Fibromyalgia

Fibromyalgia

An Essential Guide For Patients and Their Families

DANIEL J. WALLACE M.D.

JANICE BROCK WALLACE

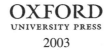

OXFORD
UNIVERSITY PRESS
2003

OXFORD

UNIVERSITY PRESS

Oxford   New York
Auckland   Bangkok   Buenos Aires   Cape Town   Chennai
Dar es Salaam   Delhi   Hong Kong   Istanbul   Karachi   Kolkata
Kuala Lumpur   Madrid   Melbourne   Mexico City   Mumbai   Nairobi
São Paulo   Shanghai   Singapore   Taipei   Tokyo   Toronto

and an associated company in Berlin

Published by Oxford University Press, Inc.
198 Madison Avenue, New York, New York, 10016

www.oup.com

Oxford is a registered trademark of Oxford University Press

Library of Congress Cataloging-in-Publication Data
Wallace, Daniel J. (Daniel Jeffrey), 1949–
Fibromyalgia : an essential guide for patients
and their families / Daniel J. Wallace, Janice Brock Wallace.
p.   cm.
Includes bibliographical references and index.
ISBN-13 978-0-19-514931-9
ISBN 0-19-514931-9 (pbk. alk. paper)
1. Fibromyalgia—Popular works. I. Wallace, Janice Brock. II. Title.
RC927.3 .W344 2002
616.7'4—dc 21   2002017096

9 8 7 6 5 4
Printed in the United States of America
on acid-free paper

Contents

Preface

The purpose of this book is to enable you to help yourself; to make it easier to work with your doctor and other allied health professionals; to improve the way you feel; and to promote a better quality of life. To begin, there are several reasons why fibromyalgia is plagued by misunderstanding:

■ Although it is now recognized as a legitimate syndrome by the American Medical Association, American College of Rheumatology, Arthritis Foundation, and American College of Physicians, as well as the World Health Organization, some doctors still question its existence. This is largely a consequence of incomplete medical training that was (and often still is) primarily hospital based. Outpatient (office-based) clinical medicine training, which included fibromyalgia, was largely overlooked. Patients are rarely, if ever, hospitalized for fibromyalgia. Also, statistically validated criteria for defining fibromyalgia were not endorsed by organized medicine until 1990. Many physicians are therefore unaware that fibromyalgia has been accorded its own coding number for insurance billing (7290).

■ Fibromyalgia patients often have normal blood tests and imaging studies and are thought by some healthcare professionals to make up many of their symptoms. Certain doctors consider fibromyalgia patients to be hypochondriacs or seekers of medical attention for purposes of litigation or secondary gain. Fortunately, there are now reproducible tests documenting that these complaints are real and studies showing that hypochondriasis is extremely rare in fibromyalgia.

■ Six million Americans meet the criteria for fibromyalgia. On the average, they saw an average of four doctors before they were correctly diagnosed, and many were convinced they had a life-threatening illness such as a body-wide cancer. Fibromyalgia is a combination of pain, fatigue, and systemic symptoms. Ten million patient visits to doctors every year in the United States are for pain; $85 billion is spent annually to diagnose or manage chronic pain, including litigation fees. One group has estimated that patients with fibromyalgia run up $14 billion in medical expenses annually. Additionally, at any visit, 15 percent of all patients tell their doctors they are tired. There is a paucity of reliable, detailed information about the fibromyalgia syndrome that patients can use to help themselves or others.

■ Many employers do not realize that fibromyalgia is a treatable workplace problem. It can impair job performance even though its symptoms and signs are invisible. Overall, 700 million work days are lost annually due to pain and 50 million Americans are partially disabled due to chronic pain. Up to 10 percent of fibromyalgia patients are totally disabled, 30 percent require job modifications, and 30 percent have to change their jobs in order to remain employed. Appropriate treatment, workstation modifications, and counseling could save the American public hundreds of millions of dollars, improve our productivity, and maintain the self-esteem of the fibromyalgia sufferer.

■ Every year, $13 billion is spent out of pocket for non-insurance-reimbursed care by alternative medicine physicians and other caregivers in the United States. Some of this is spent by fibromyalgia patients who are frustrated by the lack of attention, knowledge, and concern of their primary care and specialist physicians.

■ In our opinion, there is a relative shortage of rheumatologists, the subspecialists within internal medicine who deal with fibromyalgia, and too little research is ongoing to understand its cause, diagnosis, and treatment. In 2000, the National Institutes of Health allocated only $1 million for fibromyalgia research.

This book is intended not only for fibromyalgia patients, but also for their loved ones, primary care physicians, allied health professionals (nurses, social workers, dentists, physical therapists, psychologists, occupational therapists, vocational rehabilitation counselors, physician assistants, chiropractors, and dietitians), and other people who care about them.

Since the original iteration of this concept, originally published as *Making Sense of Fibromyalgia*, was written five years ago, many advances have been made in fibromyalogy. Thus, this effort has been renamed. *All About Fibromyalgia* includes over 500 changes and 20 new sections. This effort, *A Short Guide to Fibromyalgia* is a more concise, less basic-science-oriented companion volume. We gratefully acknowledge the assistance provided us by Joan Bossert of Oxford University Press, the Arthritis Foundation's Southern California Chapter (especially Lori Port and James Louie, M.D.), Dr. Allan Metzger, Frances Brock, Terri Hoffman for her artwork, and our children, Naomi, Phillip, and Sarah.

Daniel and Janice Wallace
Los Angeles, California
July, 2002

Fibromyalgia

1
What Is Fibromyalgia?

If you have the chronic pain of fibromyalgia, you may be frustrated by the lack of understanding shown by people around you. This is particularly true of the people you live and work with. If only they could feel for one day how you feel all year! Pain has no memory and no mercy. Is it like a bad flu or a severe headache? How can you find the words to describe it?

When the Arthritis Foundation tried to categorize the 150 different forms of musculoskeletal conditions in 1963, it created a classification known as *soft tissue rheumatism.* Included in this listing are conditions in which joints are *not* involved. Soft tissue rheumatism encompasses the supporting structures of joints (e.g., ligaments, bursae, and tendons), muscles, and other soft tissues. Fibromyalgia is a form of soft tissue rheumatism. A combination of three terms—fibro- (from the Latin *fibra,* or fibrous tissue), *myo-* (the Greek prefix *myos,* for muscles), and algia (from the Greek *algos,* which denotes pain)— fibromyalgia replaces earlier names for the syndrome that are still used by doctors and other health professionals such as *myofibrositis, myofascitis, muscular rheumatism, fibrositis,* and *generalized musculoligamenous strain.* Fibromyalgia is *not* a form of arthritis, since it is not associated with joint inflammation.

HOW OUR UNDERSTANDING OF FIBROMYALGIA EVOLVED

Evidence for the syndrome can be found as far back in history as the book of Job, where he complained of "sinews [that] take no rest." Seemingly exaggerated tenderness of the muscles and soft tissues to touch was documented in the nineteenth-century medical literature by French, German, and British scientists, who called it *spinal irritation, Charcot's hysteria,* or a *morbid affection.* The English physician Sir William Gowers (1845–1915) coined the term *fibrositis* in 1904 in a paper on lumbago (low back pain) when he tried to describe inflammatory changes in the fibrous tissues of the muscles of the low back. Gowers was wrong. There is no such thing as inflammation of the fibrous tissues, but the term lived on because British physicians used *fibrositis* to denote pain in the upper back and neck areas among Welsh coal miners in the 1920s and 1930s. The definition of fibrositis cross-pollinated during the Second World War when United States, Canadian, Australian, and New Zealand physicians served with their British counterparts. Soldiers who were unwilling to fight or who experienced shell shock, or complained of aches and pains due to carrying heavy gear without any obvious disease, were diagnosed as having fibrositis. Rheumatology established its first fellowship and training programs in the United States after World War II and, more often than not, their directors were medical officers who had become interested in the discipline as a result of working with their British colleagues. No substantive changes in the understanding of fibrositis were evident until a series of very important observations were published by the rheumatologist Hugh Smythe and his colleagues at the University of Toronto in the mid-1970s. They renamed the disorder *"fibrositis syndrome"* and convincingly connected it to systemic symptoms such as fatigue and sleep abnormalities. Smythe popularized the use of the *tender point examination* suggested by others and frequently referred to fibrositis as a *pain amplification disorder.*

Smythe's connection of fibrositis with systemic symptoms and the inappropriateness of the term *fibrositis* (since no inflammation was present) prompted Dr. Muhammed Yunus and his associates at the University of Illinois at Peoria to take up a suggestion of Dr. Kahler Hench (son of Dr. Phillip Hench, the only rheumatologist to win a Nobel Prize for discovering that cortisone helped arthritis) that the term *fibromyalgia* better described the syndrome. Yunus was also the first to validate statistically the benefits of measuring tender points and to compare fibromyalgia populations with healthy, normal, or control groups. Published in 1981, these observations were immediately endorsed by nearly all rheumatologists. Yunus also was the first investigator to associate objectively what is now called *chronic neuromuscular pain* complaints such as irritable colon, tension headache, numbness, tingling, and swelling or edema with the disorder. He also postulated that chemicals creating these symptoms and signs are also influenced by factors such as emotional or physical stress or trauma, mood, and behavior.

During the 1980s, studies showed that patients diagnosed with fibromyalgia included many originally described as having conditions such as muscular rheumatism, musculoligamentous strain, and other syndromes diagnosed by orthopedists, neurologists, neurosurgeons, and physical medicine specialists. Further, the development of tests supporting scientifically acceptable, reproducible abnormalities in fibromyalgia led the American Medical Association in 1987 to editorialize that the syndrome truly existed. A committee subsequently was formed to devise a definition and description of fibromyalgia for statistical and research purposes, and these criteria were adopted by the American College of Rheumatology in 1990.

THE AMERICAN COLLEGE OF RHEUMATOLOGY (ACR) FIBROMYALGIA CRITERIA

In the late 1980s, a Multicenter Criteria Committee under the direction of Dr. Frederick Wolfe at the University of Kansas was formed to define fibromyalgia. Patient groups were evaluated for a variety of symptoms, signs, and laboratory abnormalities in an effort to ascertain which factors were the most *sensitive* and *specific* for defining the disorder. In other words, the investigators wanted to identify the most frequently found features of fibromyalgia (sensitivity) that could help doctors differentiate it from other disorders (specificity). The list in Table 1 (illustrated in Fig. 1) was 88.4 percent sensitive and 81.1 percent specific in identifying fibromyalgia patients. As a result, these criteria were endorsed in 1990 by the American College of Rheumatology (ACR), the association to which nearly all 5,000 rheumatologists in the United States and Canada belong. Focusing in Table 1 and Figure 1, fibromyalgia essentially is:

1. Widespread pain of at least 3 months' duration (this rules out viruses or traumatic insults that resolve on their own).

2. Pain in all four quadrants of the body (picture cutting the body into quarters, as in a pie): right side, left side, above the waist, below the waist.
3. Pain occurring in at least 11 of 18 specified "tender" points (as shown in the figure) with at least one point in each quadrant.
4. Pain defined, in this context, as discomfort when 8 pounds of pressure are applied to the tender point.
5. Tender points usually occur in a specific distribution. For instance, 8 of the 18 tender points are in the upper back and neck area, and only 2 are below the buttocks. The reader should be aware that tender points can occur almost anywhere in the body; the ACR criteria simply represent the most common 18 points.

Once fibromyalgia was defined, it was possible to perform more reliable studies on this syndrome, since all researchers would use the same definition. We could now explore how many people in the United States had fibromyalgia, determine what their primary complaints were, and identify groups of people on whom to test new treatments.

How do certain symptoms and signs fibromyalgia is associated with such as fatigue, sleep disturbances, and bowel complaints, fit into the definition of fibromyalgia? A group of international fibromyalgia experts issued what was termed the Copenhagen Declaration in 1992 and adopted by the World Health Organization in 1993. They recognized the use of the ACR criteria for research purposes but defined fibromyalgia as being part of a wider spectrum encompassing headache, irritable bladder, spastic colitis, painful menstrual periods, temperature sensitivity, atypical patterns of numbness and tingling, exercise intolerance, and complaints of weakness in addition to persistent fatigue, stiffness, and nonrestoring sleep.

FIBROMYALGIA TERMINOLOGY: CLASSIFICATION AND REGIONAL FORMS

Many rheumatologists recognize two types of fibromyalgia: primary and secondary. The cause of *primary fibromyalgia syndrome* is unknown, but it can be induced by trauma, infection, stress, inflammation, or other factors. *Secondary fibromyalgia* occurs when a primary

Table 1. *The 1990 ACR criteria for fibromyalgia*

1. *History of widespread pain.*

   Definition: Pain is considered widespread when all of the following are present: pain in the left side of the body, pain in the right side of the body, pain above the waist and pain below the waist. In addition, axial skeletal pain (cervical spine or anterior chest or thoracic spine or low back) must be present. In this definition shoulder and buttock pain is considered as pain for each involved side. "Low back" pain is considered lower segment pain.

2. *Pain in 11 of 18 tender point sites on digital palpation.*

   Definition: Pain, on digital palpation, must be present in at least 11 of the following 18 tender point sites:

   Occiput: bilateral, at the suboccipital muscle insertions.

   Low cervical: bilateral, at the anterior aspects of the inter-transverse spaces at C5–C7.

   Trapezius: bilateral, at the midpoint of the upper border.

   Supraspinatus: bilateral, at origins, above the scapula spine near the medial border.

   2nd rib: bilateral, at the second costochondral junctions, just lateral to the junctions on upper surfaces.

   Lateral epicondyle: bilateral, 2 cm distal to the epicondyles.

   Gluteal: bilateral, in upper outer quadrants of buttocks in anterior fold of muscle.

   Greater trochanter: bilateral, posterior to the trochanteric prominence.

   Knees: bilateral, at the medial fat pad proximal to the joint line.

   For a tender point to be considered "positive" the subject must state that the palpation was painful. "Tender" is not to be considered painful.

Note: For classification purposes patients will be said to have fibromyalgia if both criteria are satisfied. Widespread pain must have been present for at least 3 months. The presence of a second clinical disorder does not exclude the diagnosis of fibromyalgia.

condition, such as hypothyroidism or lupus, creates a concomitant fibromyalgia, the treatment of which may make the syndrome disappear. Sometimes, pain identical to that associated with fibromyalgia is located in specific areas or regions or in one quadrant of the body. For example, patients may have jaw and neck pain on one side and no discomfort anywhere else. Regional forms of fibromyalgia are called *regional myofascial syndrome* or *myofascial pain syndrome*.

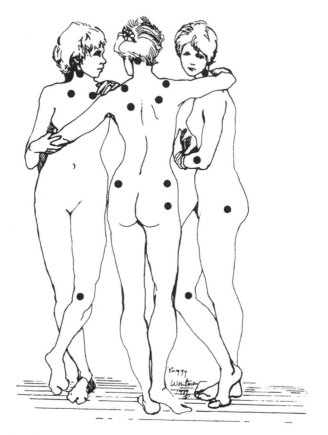

Fig. 1 *Fibromyalgia tender points. (Adapted from "The Three Graces,"*
Louvre Museum, Paris. From D.J. Wallace, The Lupus Book.
New York: Oxford University Press, 1995, p. 170; reprinted with
permission from Dr. F. Wolfe.)

Finally, patients may hear a lot about trigger points or tender points.
Many doctors consider them to be the same thing. However, for research purposes, there are subtle differences. A *tender point* is an area
of tenderness in the muscles, tendons, bony prominences, or fat pads,
whereas a *trigger point* shoots down to another area. For instance,
when a trigger point is touched, it shoots pain to other muscles. Like
pulling a trigger in a gun, it sends out a bullet that travels, and pain can
be felt in areas away from the trigger.

HOW TO RESPOND TO PEOPLE WHO DO NOT BELIEVE FIBROMYALGIA EXISTS

Since fibromyalgia is a relatively new entity, some physicians who may have had the topic barely covered in medical school tend to downplay its importance, say "it's all psychiatric," or deny its existence. Many training programs are almost entirely hospital based and few patients with fibromyalgia are ever hospitalized for it. Most importantly, fibromyalgia is not a *disease*, it is a *syndrome* or a *construct*. Simply stated, fibromyalgia is a form of *chronic neuromuscular pain* that meets statistically validated criteria. Some doctors don't like the name *fibromyalgia* because it could stigmatize patients. Since the syndrome encompasses individuals with lupus, scoliosis, and hypothyroidism, fibromyalgia's boundaries tend to defy the occasional patient's desire to blame the syndrome as the reason why they cannot work, function in society, or be happy. The authors have heard fibromyalgia being called *the emperor's new clothes syndrome, generalized rheumatism*, or *feeling out of sorts*. Nevertheless, every recognized medical organization from the American College of Rheumatology, the American Medical Association, World Health Organization, and the American College of Physicians to medical insurers have endorsed its existence. There has never been a published peer-review study or report from a medical society challenging the validity of fibromyalgia as a syndrome or construct. Finally, some critics refuse to recognize fibromyalgia as an entity because it lacks firm physical signs. Not only is this not the case, but the same analogy applies to migraine headaches. Nobody disputes the existence of migraines, and Americans spend $14 billion a year on its treatment.

SUMMING UP

The term *fibromyalgia* refers to a complex syndrome characterized by pain amplification, musculoskeletal discomfort, and systemic symptoms. Although its existence was questioned in the past, nearly all rheumatologists, medical societies, and the overwhelming majority of physicians now accept fibromyalgia as a distinct diagnostic entity.

2

Who Gets Fibromyalgia
and Why?

HOW PREVALENT IS FIBROMYALGIA?

Until recently, nobody knew how many people had fibromyalgia. Several surveys suggest that while 2 percent of the adult U.S. population have full-blown fibromyalgia (3.5 percent of adult women and 0.5 percent of adult men), 11 percent have chronic widespread pain and 20 percent have chronic regional pain. Recently, Dr. Larry Bradley at the University of Alabama has found that for every diagnosed fibromyalgia patient in the United States, there is an undiagnosed individual who has the requisite tender points, but never seeks medical attention for this. This has been termed *community fibromyalgia*. A survey in Great Britain found that 13 percent of the population had chronic widespread pain, 72 percent of whom sought medical attention for it. Of those, 21 percent fulfilled the ACR criteria for fibromyalgia. In other words, of individuals with chronic neuromuscular pain, less than half have diagnosed fibromyalgia or community fibromyalgia.

Fibromyalgia is the third or fourth most common reason for consulting a rheumatologist. Approximately 15–20 percent of all patients seeking rheumatology referrals have fibromyalgia. The 5,000 rheumatologists in the United States who are trained in internal medicine and subspecialize in managing more than 150 musculoskeletal and immune system disorders are very familiar with the diagnosis and treatment of fibromyalgia.

WHO DEVELOPS FIBROMYALGIA?

Even though 1 American in 50 has fibromyalgia, the syndrome is distributed unevenly across the population, meaning 80–90 percent of patients with the condition are women. (One theory contends that women have a lower pain threshold than men, which is hormonally related.) Fibromyalgia is extremely uncommon in children and rarely appears for the first time in older persons. Within these groups, complaints and clinical features are atypical. In the United States, fibromyalgia is more common among Caucasians than among other racial groups. Using the ACR criteria or other earlier suggested criteria, the prevalence of fibromyalgia in other countries or regions (mostly in Europe, Canada, and Australia) has ranged from 0.5 percent to 12 percent.

Are humans the only species to develop fibromyalgia? Probably not. Lameness has been observed in dogs for some time, and articles in the veterinary literature convincingly show that they can also have tender points.

Most of our fibromyalgia patients are in their prime of life and at the peaks of their careers. Surveys have shown that most patients develop the syndrome in their 30s and 40s. Fibromyalgia infrequently evolves during adolescence. Whereas 60 percent of cases are diagnosed in people between the ages of 30 and 49, another 35 percent of patients are diagnosed in their 20s or between the ages of 50 and 65. The reasons for this distribution are not clear, but the decline in onset after the age of 50 may have something to do with menopause in women, which may alleviate (but occasionally aggravate) certain fibromyalgia symptoms.

IS FIBROMYALGIA GENETIC?

Even though no fibromyalgia genetic markers have been found, we are aware of studies documenting a high prevalence of the syndrome among certain families. For example, in one well documented study, 28 percent of children of fibromyalgia patients ultimately developed the syndrome. Whether this is due to a yet-undiscovered genetic marker or markers, or from environmental or psychological factors is still unclear. Recently, Dr. Yunus has conducted studies suggesting that pain amplification may be genetically mediated. Serotonin is a chemical that can help diminish pain. Recently, scientists have found several genetically determined variants of serotonin. Whether this results in people having different perceptions of pain is not known.

WHAT ARE SOME OF THE CAUSES
OF FIBROMYALGIA?

What turns on the fibromyalgia syndrome? When we ask patients what they feel caused their fibromyalgia, trauma, infections, and stress are the three most common responses.

Fibromyalgia Resulting from a Single-Event Trauma

When we last counted, there were 47 different reported secondary causes of fibromyalgia. *According to patients,* the most common cause of secondary fibromyalgia is trauma. There are two types of trauma: injury resulting from a single event or continuous trauma with resulting repetitive injury.

First, let's discuss a single-event injury. Suppose that in your community 100 people sustain a whiplash injury from a 10-mile-per-hour rear-ender automobile accident on a given day. Whiplash, a term coined by H.D. Crowe in 1928, is the only diagnosis relating to causation rather than the tissue involved. A whiplash injury occurs when a car driver or passenger is rear-ended. The head and neck stay still at first, while the body jerks forward. As the body returns back, the neck hyperextends backward. What happens to people after a whiplash injury? Many will go to their doctors within days and report pain in their upper back and neck areas. Their doctors will prescribe ibuprofen or naproxen-like anti-inflammatory agents, a muscle relaxant, and perhaps even a small prescription for a strong pain killer. A minority may be given neck collars or physical or chiropractic therapy. After two to three months, all but 2–5 percent (up to 21 percent in some studies) of the patients will get better and gradually discontinue all therapy. But what about the remaining people? Strange things start to happen. For completely unclear reasons, these 2–5 percent begin to hurt more and their pain becomes widespread. They complain of lower back and leg pain (areas that were not injured), begin noticing difficulty sleeping, and become fatigued. Ultimately, they are diagnosed as having fibromyalgia. Many doctors don't understand this; they suffered the same trivial injury with the same impact from which other patients fully recover! We have seen this with slip-and-fall injuries and other forms of minor trauma. This phenomenon is poorly documented in the medical literature, and since litigation frequently is involved, many doctors feel it is overdiagnosed.

Dr. Buskila and his colleagues in Israel followed 102 patients who experienced a serious whiplash injury and compared them with 59 patients who sustained leg fractures. The neck injury group was 13 times more likely to develop fibromyalgia two years later (21 percent vs. 1.7 percent), which was statistically significant. None of the few surveys cited as challenging this contention specifically looked for the diagnosis of fibromyalgia or reviewed patient charts prior to injury. From a physics standpoint, a whiplash response requires a rear-end impact of at least 8 kilometers per hour (5 miles per hour). It could thus induce fibromyalgia by creating a post-injury sleep disturbance, acting as a source of referral pain elsewhere in the body, or through a concept known as neuroplasticity. All told, about 25 percent of patients relate their fibromyalgia to trauma, but the actual incidence is much less. The diagnosis of post-traumatic fibromyalgia also varies according to who is taking care of the patient. In a Canadian study, 83 percent of rheumatologists but only 29 percent of orthopedists treating the same patients after an injury diagnosed them as having fibromyalgia. Indeed, when we look through medical records of many patients who claim their symptoms and signs of fibromyalgia resulted from an accident or trauma, there is often evidence for a pre-existing community fibromyalgia (reviewed earlier in this chapter) or a fibromyalgia-associated condition. Many whiplash-like injuries flare pre-injury fibromyalgia related complaints for several weeks to months. Prolonged flares that are claimed to be soley due to specific incidents make no physiologic sense unless they were associated with serious injuries such as fractures or newly herniated cervical discs.

Fibromyalgia from Continuous Trauma

Repetitive trauma from poor workstation body mechanics (usually associated with regional myofascial syndrome) is especially common among workers who do heavy lifting, as is reviewed in Chapter 11. The legal term *continuous trauma* opens up another can of worms because it also involves litigation, particularly worker's compensation.

What about Infections?

One of the most common self-reported causes of fibromyalgia is an infectious process, possibly a viral (e.g., an Epstein-Barr-like) illness characterized by fever, swollen glands, sore throat, and cough. When these conditions disappear, the patient develops profound aching and fatigue. Over 40 microbes have been associated with postinfectious fatigue syndromes. The inciting organisms are quite diverse and include parvovirus, the herpesvirus causing mononucleosis and Epstein-Barr, mycoplasma, *Toxoplasma gondii,* hepatitis A virus, cytomegalovirus, *Brucella,* poliovirus, the virus causing AIDS, and the bacterium causing Lyme disease.

Can Emotional Stress Cause Fibromyalgia?

Severe emotional stress or trauma frequently triggers and aggravates fibromyalgia. There is little doubt that fibromyalgia can come about or be accelerated by a diminished ability to cope with life's stresses and

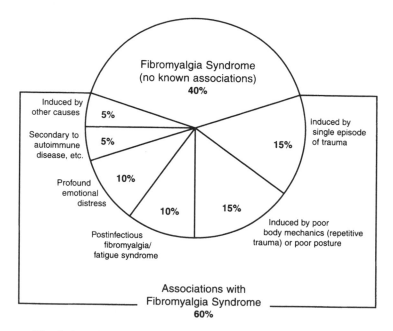

Fig. 2 *Distribution of fibromyalgia syndrome in the United States.*

traumas. How does this happen? Later sections of this book will survey models of stress that have been studied with regard to our hypothalamic-pituitary-adrenal (or stress-hormone) axis and how this relates to fibromyalgia.

Associations with Fibromyalgia

Forty percent of fibromyalgia cases appear spontaneously, and no obvious inciting factor is ever found. This condition is termed *primary fibromyalgia syndrome.* It is united by core features (widespread musculoskeletal pain and tender points), characteristic features (fatigue, stiffness, sleep disorder), and associated features (anxiety, depression, numbness, irritable bowel), and no specific inciting event is associated with its onset.

Other triggers of fibromyalgia include autoimmune diseases, withdrawal from medications (especially steroids), prescription of other medications (such as interferons), and hormonal abnormalities (particularly low thyroid level). Figure 2 shows some of the associations with fibromyalgia.

3

The Basic Science of Fibromyalgia

In this chapter, we'll explore what makes fibromyalgia a pain amplification syndrome. Why does the patient hurt in places where there was often no injury and all laboratory tests are normal? What creates what doctors call *allodynia,* or a clinical situation that results in pain from a stimulus (such as light touch) that normally should *not* be painful? Fibromyalgia is a form of chronic, widespread allodynia, as well as sustained *hyperalgesia,* or greater sensitivity than would be expected to an adverse stimulus.

NORMAL PAIN PATHWAYS

The nervous system consists of several components. The brain and spinal cord comprise the *central nervous system.* Nerves leaving the spinal cord that tell us to move our arms or legs are part of the "motor" aspects of the *peripheral nervous system.* Additionally, all sorts of information about touch, taste, chemicals, and pressure are relayed through "sensory" pathways back to the spinal cord, where they are processed and sent up to the brain for a response. The *autonomic nervous system* consists of specialized peripheral nerves. Fibromyalgia is characterized by an inappropriate neuromuscular reaction that leads to chronic pain. Patients with fibromyalgia usually react normally to acute pain.

To elaborate upon this, nerve wires from the skin, muscles, or joints send sensory signals (e.g., touch, pressure) to the spinal cord. Several separate sensory pathways have been described. The particular sensory trail important in fibromyalgia is one termed *nociception.* A *nociceptor* is a receptor that is sensitive to a noxious stimulus. Nociceptors are present in blood vessel walls, muscle, fascia, tendons, joint capsules, fat pads, and on body surfaces. A noxious stimulus can be thermal (heat, cold), mechanical (touch, pressure), or chemical. Normally, the body transmits these nociceptive impulses neurochemically from the periphery to the central nervous system. *One factor that distinguishes acute from chronic pain is that the perception of chronic pain is significantly influenced by the interaction of physiologic, psychological, and social processes.* Unlike patients with acute pain, those with chronic pain often don't appear to be in pain. Figure 3 illustrates normal nociceptive processes.

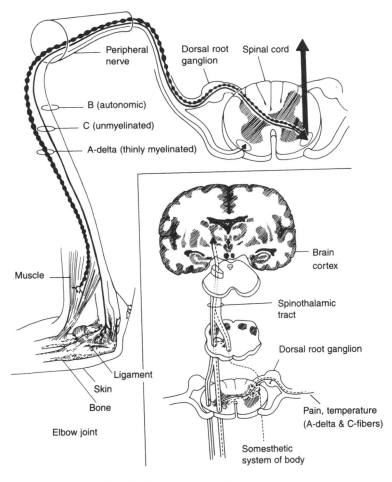

Fig. 3 *Normal nociceptive processes.*

ORGANIC PAIN: LOCALIZED VERSUS CENTRAL PAIN; NOCICEPTIVE VERSUS NEUROPATHIC PAIN

Chronic pain can be *organic* (real) or *psychogenic,* in which cases patients think their pain is physical. Organic sources of pain can be either *peripheral* or *central.* Peripheral pain results in muscular discomfort from local tender points. For instance, local injections of anesthetics such as Novocaine or xylocaine can temporarily abolish pain at a specific site. Exercising a muscle can lead to pain in that muscle.

On the other hand, pain can emanate from brain and spinal cord pathways without any peripheral tissue or nociceptive input or stimulus. A classical example is something doctors call *phantom limb* pain. Let us say that a patient has had a leg amputated below the left knee but complains that the left ankle hurts. This seems impossible, but it happens all the time. This is due to a phenomenon known as *neuroplasticity*, in which the brain has the adaptive capability to modify structure or function by growing nerve fibers, activating previously quiet nerves, or creating hypersensitization.

Table 2. *Pain classifications relevant to fibromyalgia*

I. Acute pain—usually reacts normally in fibromyalgia
II. Chronic pain
    A. Psychogenic pain—not part of fibromyalgia
    B. Organic pain
       1. Location
          a. Localized—observed in regional myofascial pain
          b. Central—observed in fibromyalgia
       2. Source
          a. Neuropathic—not part of fibromyalgia; due to damaged or injured nerves, as in diabetes, trauma, and herinated disc
          b. Nociceptive—includes features of fibromyalgia (see Glossary for definitions)
             (i) Hyperalgesia
             (ii) Neuroplasticity
             (iii) Hyperpathia
             (iv) Causalgia
          c. Non-nociceptive (allodynia)—can function as nociceptive fibers with chronic stimulation in fibromyalgia

Finally, chronic organic pain is either *nociceptive,* as in fibromyalgia, nonnociceptive, or *neuropathic.* Nociceptive pain occurs with chronic, repeated stimulation and can potentially produce tissue damage. In this circumstance, nonnociceptive fibers can act as nociceptive ones. Neuropathic pain results from a direct nerve injury that leads to nervous system dysfunction. Examples of neuropathic pain include diabetes, trauma, and herniated disc. These concepts are summarized in Table 2. *Hyperalgesia* is an exaggerated response to a painful stimulus. Inappropriately increased hyperalgesia results when repeated stimuli from areas within tissues lower the thresholds for activating nociceptors. As a result, seemingly innocuous stimuli such as light touching can cause severe pain.

The mechanism or mechanisms that cause(s) nociceptive pain loops to amplify pain rather than suppress pain in fibromyalgia is the subject of numerous ongoing studies. A summary of what goes awry in fibromyalgia will now be reviewed.

WHAT CAUSES "PAIN WITHOUT PURPOSE?"

Small C-fibers in the skin are easily activated by chemical, mechanical or thermal energy. Even without noxious stimuli, signals can arise spontaneously that are converted into neural impulses. Once sensitized by an inciting stimulus, various signals are sent through C-fiber nerves to the dorsal root ganglion of the spinal cord. If there are too many incoming signals, the spinal cord can have a hard time sorting them out and filtering them. The constant bombardment of noxious inputs by C-fibers leads to *central sensitization* (central refers to the spinal cord) and produces a *wind-up* phenomenon. During the wind-up process, pain is enhanced by each painful or nonpainful stimulus. Large A-delta fibers, which usually only transmit very noxious impulses, start carrying some of the signals usually carried by the C-fibers. Light touch is thus misinterpreted by the spinal cord and brain as hyperalgesia. Even the autonomic B-fibers start carrying nociceptive stimuli to handle the overload. At this point, nonnociceptive fibers start to carry nociceptive signals. Known as allodynia, its maintenance becomes dependent upon continued central sensitization. In the dorsal root ganglion, increased discharges of second- and third-rung neurons in response to repetitive C-fiber stimulation takes place. This long-term hyperexcitability leads to a lower firing threshold and expansion of receptor fields, which are dependent upon size, location, electrical thresholds for firing, and selectivity of the receptor. All this is accomplished through neurochemicals. Nociceptive signals cause the secretion of nerve growth factor that produces a chemical known as substance P (for pain). Substance P facilitates nociception by altering spinal cord neurons (nerve cells) to respond to incoming nociceptive peripheral signals. It migrates up and down the spinal cord, which ultimately leads to the generalization of fibromyalgia pain to other areas. Substance P turns on NMDA receptors. *NMDA receptors (N-methyl-D-aspartate)* are usually dormant and play no role in acute pain. Enhanced electrical depolarization causes calcium influx into nerve cells that makes them more excitable. NMDA-related signals ascend to the brain and are processed in the thalamus (and B-fibers in the limbic system).

The brain is now ready to meet this challenge by the inhibitory actions of neurotransmitters in the descending system. However, in fibromyalgia, serotonin levels are relatively low, which further causes more substance P to be made—this time in the brain. To clarify these complicated actions, we will now elaborate upon some of the chemicals we mentioned (and others) in more detail. These are shown in Figure 4.

WHAT'S WRONG WITH MY MUSCLES?

Since most fibromyalgia patients complain of aching and spasm in their muscles, common sense suggests that there must be something wrong with the muscle. Our bodies have 640 different muscles, which constitute as much as 40 percent of our weight. When physicians look at the muscles of fibromyalgia patients under a simple microscope, they generally appear normal. In fact, muscles must be looked at under an electron microscope (which magnifies the tissue thousands of times) in order to find any consistent abnormalities. In this setting there are subtle alterations, including the deposition of a chemical, glycogen, swollen, and abnormal cell organelles known as mitochondria, increased DNA fragmentation, ragged red fibers, and smeared muscle cell membranes. Some investigators have shown that magnesium levels are low

CHRONIC PAIN PATHWAYS IN FIBROMYALGIA

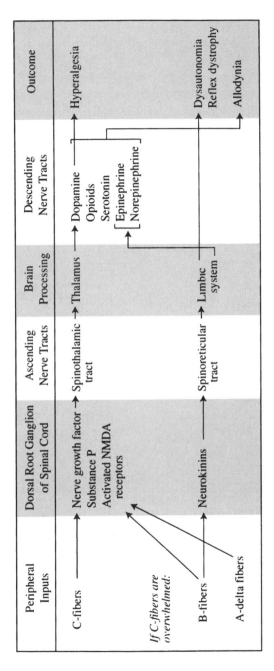

Fig. 4 *Pain pathways important to fibromyalgia.*

in the muscles of fibromyalgia patients. Fibromyalgia patients are generally deconditioned. In other words, they are out of shape. Of course, many more people are out of shape than have fibromyalgia, but studies of muscles from out-of-shape people also show some of these alterations.

Electrical activity in muscles can be assessed by an electromyogram (EMG). This "cardiogram of the muscles" also is normal when performed conventionally. However, if the EMG is performed with special maneuvers not usually performed with standard testing, fibromyalgic muscles may have difficulty relaxing after exertion and, when they are deprived of oxygen, have more spontaneous electrical activity.

Microtrauma and "Taut Bands"

When healthy but sedentary people exert themselves abnormally, such as on a ski or hiking trip, this unaccustomed exertion results in muscle soreness and stiffness. Some of this pain could be due to microscopic

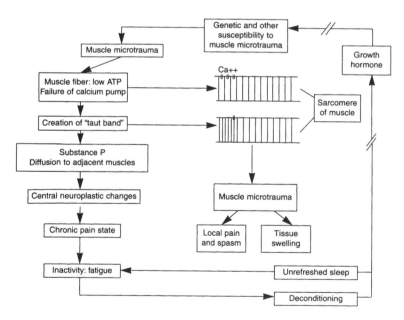

Fig. 5 *The muscle in fibromyalgia. Microtrauma creates a sequence of events leading to muscle spasm and not enough oxygen getting to muscles, which produces pain.*

muscle tears resulting in leakage of chemicals that produce discomfort. This usually lasts a day or two, and then the body's repair mechanisms take care of the problem. In fibromyalgia, the soreness and stiffness become chronic. How does this happen? Follow the sequences illustrated in Figure 5 as we describe this hypothesis.

When a focal injury affects a muscle fiber, it contains both relaxed and contracted units, or sarcomeres. This causes potassium to leave muscles and sarcomeres to stimulate Type C unmyelinated pain nerve endings. The ensuing hyperexcitability of spinal cord neurons sensitizes second order neurons. Nonnociceptive impulses produce allodynia, and nociceptive impulses hyperalgesia. In turn, a calcium-ATP (or energy) pump is activated, unleashing events that produce a *taut band*. In other words, some of the muscle becomes as tight as a rubber band, while adjacent muscle relaxes. As a result of this chain of events, insufficient oxygen reaches muscles. Additionally, there are focal decreases in critical muscle enzyme levels that provide energy and fuel, as well as the release of substance P to nearby sarcomeres, producing pain and spasm. Some of these chemicals sensitize the nervous system, which perpetuates the vicious cycle of pain and spasm. Also, growth hormone and its liver by-product, insulin-like growth factor 1 (IGF-1), are made during deep sleep and promote repair of muscles damaged by microtrauma. When patients sleep poorly, this repair is interfered with. Tender points occur at muscle-tendon junctions, where mechanical forces produce the most injury.

Muscles: Summing Up

Although muscles usually look normal in fibromyalgia, and although many of the changes described in muscle tissues reflect being out of shape, there are probably certain unique self-perpetuating events that produce muscle pain and spasm through the interplay of microtrauma, pain, chemicals, and unrefreshing sleep.

STRESS AND THE HPA AXIS

Within the brain is a small region known as the *hypothalamus*. It makes releasing hormones that travel down a short path to the pituitary gland, which makes stimulating hormones. The stimulating hormones send signals to tissues where hormones are manufactured for specialized functions. Table 3 shows how thyroid, cortisol, insulin, breast milk, and growth hormone are made along the hypothalamic-pituitary axis and the hypothalamic-pituitary-adrenal (HPA) axis.

We have already mentioned that emotional stress can bring on or aggravate fibromyalgia. The role of corticotropin-releasing hormone (CRH), the precursor or ancestor of the steroid known as *cortisol,* has been the focus of much of this work. Even though CRH levels are normal in fibromyalgia, CRH responses (stress responses) to different forms of stimulation are blunted. How do these interrelationships translate into a fibromyalgia patient's feeling of being unwell? The answer is not clear. However, these studies suggest that fibromyalgia patients do not respond normally to acute stress and do not release enough adrenalin. This leads to a chronic stress state to which the body reacts by making things worse, creating a vicious cycle that perpetuates the unwell feeling.

Table 3. *Important hormones derived from the hypothalamic-pituitary axis*

Hypothalamus (Releasers)	Pituitary (Stimulators)	Peripheral tissues (Hormones)
Corticotropin-releasing hormone (CRH)	Adrenocorticortropic hormone (ACTH)	Cortisone
Thyrotropin-releasing hormone (TRH)	Thyroid-stimulating hormone (TSH)	Thyroid
Growth hormone–releasing hormone	Growth hormone (GH)	
Prolactin-releasing factor (PRF)	Prolactin	Breast milk
Gonadotropin-releasing hormone (GnRH)	Follicle-stimulating hormone, luteinizing hormone (FSH, LH)	Estrogen, progesterone

SLEEP, HORMONES, AND FIBROMYALGIA

Somewhere between 60 and 90 percent of fibromyalgia patients have difficulty sleeping. They might be in bed for eight hours but do not wake up feeling refreshed, a condition termed *nonrestorative sleep.* Work done by Dr. Harvey Moldofsky at the University of Toronto since the 1970s has documented sleep brain-wave abnormalities in fibromyalgia patients. If doctors attached an electroencephalograph (EEG) to the scalp and took a "cardiogram" of the brain of a sleeping healthy person, they would find four phases of sleep. Most of the time is taken up by a deep *slow-wave sleep,* characterized by delta waves on the electrical tracing. Approximately 20 percent of sleep time is spent dreaming, which is termed *rapid eye movement* (REM) sleep. The majority of fibromyalgia patients have alpha waves (which should not be there) intruding into delta-wave sleep, compared with only 10–15 percent of persons without the syndrome. Alpha-delta intrusion can have a startle effect and awaken the person. Sometimes, it may cause one to turn over, shake a leg, grit the teeth, or open the eyes. After a while, it keeps one from falling into a deep sleep. Some fibromyalgia patients have alpha-delta intrusion hundreds of times during an evening. It's no wonder that they wake up feeling more tired than before they went to sleep!

Even fully grown adults require growth hormone for a variety of purposes. Most growth hormone is produced when we are in slow (delta) wave sleep. Levels of a product of growth hormone known as IGF-1 (insulin-like growth factor) are decreased by 30 percent in fibromyalgia, especially in the early morning. CRH also promotes the release of a chemical that blocks growth hormone secretion. Dr. Robert Bennett at the University of Oregon has theorized that the low levels of growth hormone observed in fibromyalgia patients (as measured by their by-products, IGF) make them more susceptible to muscle trauma because micro-trauma occurring during the day cannot be repaired at night. Patients with low growth hormone levels have decreased energy, exercise capacity muscle weakness, and impaired cognition.

What does this mean in a practical sense? Abnormal electrical waves keep fibromyalgia patients up at night, which, in turn, prevents enough growth hormone from being made to repair and restore their muscles. Moreover, fragmentation of sleep occurs with menstruation, stress, pain trauma, infection, or a change in the weather.

CONNECTING HORMONES AND NERVES WITH THE IMMUNE SYSTEM AND CYTOKINES

What goes wrong with the immune system in fibromyalgia? When the body is attacked, the immune system comes to the rescue. We have a very sophisticated immune surveillance system, and it may come as a surprise that this system is reasonably intact in fibromyalgia. For example, in fibromyalgia studies of immune responsiveness, T-cell and B-cell counts, levels of autoantibodies (such as antinuclear antibody and rheumatoid factor), and the effectiveness of immunizations and allergy shots are usually normal. When I explain this to some patients, they ask why they develop so many infections or have lupus-like signs such as Raynaud's phenomenon (in which the fingers turn different colors in cold weather). There are explanations for this, some related to the ANS (see the next chapter) and others related to overlapping features with chronic fatigue syndrome.

One of the immune system's components involves a group of cellular protein hormones known as *cytokines*. Cytokines play a role in the growth and development of T-and B-cells and have exotic names such as *interleukins* and *interferons*. They amplify or "gear up" T-cells and B-cells, which are types of white blood cells known as *lymphocytes*. Even though cytokine blood levels are normal in patients with fibromyalgia, the administration of cytokines to treat diseases (such as alpha-interferon to manage hepatitis or interleukin-2 for advanced cancer) *induces* or causes fibromyalgia. Table 4 lists how cytokines can influence manifestations of fibromyalgia.

Figure 6 illustrates some of the disease interrelationships of hormones, sleep, and the immune system.

WHAT IS THE AUTONOMIC NERVOUS SYSTEM?

Finally, it's time to introduce a special subset of the peripheral nervous system, known as the *autonomic nervous system (ANS)*. The ANS consists of two types of fibers: sympathetic and parasympathetic. The *sympathetic nervous system (SNS)* is our "fight or flight" mechanism. It releases adrenalin when we are threatened and "revs up the juices," resulting in aggressive behavior or self-protection. The ANS also regulates our pulse and blood pressure by constricting or dilating blood

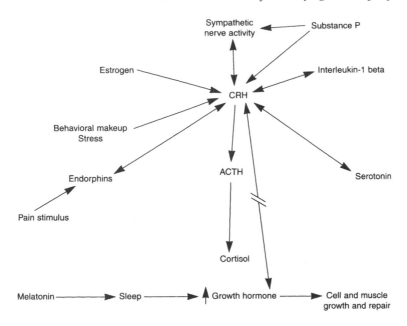

Fig. 6 *The body's "stress hormone" system. Cortisol, estrogen, pain chemicals, muscles, sleep, stress, and the ANS all interact with each other.*

vessels. Additionally, the ANS can relax or contract muscles and regulate sweat, urine, and defecation reflexes. The ability of the SNS to stimulate sensory fibers that meld into the nociceptive pathway is extremely important. At the same time that nociceptive influences are being processed and sent up the spinothalamic tract, parallel signals from B-fibers (autonomic fibers) are received and sent to the limbic system of the brain via the *spinoreticular tract.* The limbic system helps modulate many of our emotions, including alertness, vigilance, and fear.

Part of the peripheral nervous system, the ANS consists of the sympathetic nervous system (SNS), which consists of outflow from the thoracic and upper lumbar spine, and the *parasympathetic nervous system* (PNS), including outflow from the cranial nerves emanating from the upper spine and also from the mid-lumbar to the sacral areas at the buttock region. Several neurochemicals help transmit autonomic instructions. These include *epinephrine* (adrenalin), *norepinephrine* (noradrenalin), *dopamine,* and *acetylcholine.*

Table 4. *How cytokines can influence fibromyalgia*

Cytokine	Association
IL-1 beta	hyperalgesia, fatigue, sleep, muscle aches, blocks substance P
IL-2	muscle aches, cognitive dysfunction
IL-6	fatigue, hyperalgesia, depression, activates sympathetic nervous system
IL-8	production stimulated by substance P, mediates sympathetic nervous system pain
IL-10	blocks pain
TNF-alpha	produces sleep, allodynia, increases NMDA activity, regulates substance P expression

Our bodies have numerous receptors or surveillance sensors that detect heat, cold, and inflammation. These ANS sensors perform a function known as *autoregulation.* As an example of how the ANS normally works, why don't we pass out when we suddenly jump out of bed? Because the ANS instantly constricts our blood vessels peripherally and dilates them centrally. In other words, as blood is pooled to the heart and the brain, the ANS adjusts our blood pressure and regulates our pulse, or heart rate, so that we don't collapse. On the local level, these sensors dilate or constrict flow from blood vessels. They can secondarily contract and relax muscles, open and close lung airways, or cause us to sweat. For instance, ANS sensors can tone muscles, regulate urine, and regulate bowel movements, as well as dilate or constrict our pupils. The SNS releases epinephrine and norepinephrine as well as a neurochemical called dopamine. Whereas the SNS often acts as an acute stress response, the PNS arm tends to protect and conserve body processes and resources. The SNS and PNS sometimes work at cross purposes, but frequently they work together to permit actions such as normal sexual functioning and urination.

Fibromyalgia and an Abnormally Regulated ANS

The SNS is underactive in fibromyalgia. How do the workings of the ANS relate to fibromyalgia? For example, some fibromyalgia patients have *neurally mediated hypotension* in which decreased sympathetic activity lowers blood pressure, leading to dizziness and fatigue.

According to Dr. Daniel J. Clauw at The University of Michigan, the ANS control mechanisms are out of sync in certain patients with fibromyalgia. Sensors dilate the blood vessels in one area and constrict them in an adjacent region without reason or provocation. Termed *autonomic dysregulation,* or *dysautonomia,* this loss of autoregulatory or local control causes a variety of clinical problems associated with fibromyalgia.

How do the ANS sensors lose their fine-tuning control? Autonomic signals are transmitted from the periphery by events such as physical trauma or changes in posture by myelinated B-fibers via a few detours to the spinal cord. From there the ANS ascends the spinal cord via the spinoreticular tract to the limbic system of the brain. In fibromyalgia, however, repeated incoming signals from unmyelinated C-fibers to the dorsal horn of the spinal cord may also create nociceptor hypersensitivity. Further overwhelming sympathetic controls cause autonomic B-fibers to carry messages usually carried by C-fibers. Nociceptive stimuli are now transmitted through normally nonnociceptive transmitters. This results in blood vessel constriction and hyperalgesia. When this leads to the appearance or sensation of swelling, it is called *neurogenic inflammation.* Here, sensory afferent end-organ stimuli causes SNS and neuropeptide release, which produces plasma extravasation, or swelling (edema). This swelling presses on small nerves and creates the sensation of numbness, burning, or tingling. Further, substance P can activate SNS receptors in the dorsal root ganglion.

Dysautonomia Allows Fibromyalgia to Mimic Autoimmune Diseases

Altered SNS tone can mimic immunologic or autoimmune disorders. Autoimmune disorders occur when the body becomes allergic to itself. Dysautonomia produces *reactive hyperemia,* or redness in the skin after palpation. This leads to a mottled appearance under the skin and can mimic or cause *dermatographia* (rubbing a key into the skin produces an impression that lasts for minutes), *livedo reticularis* (a red, lace-like, checkerboard appearance under the skin), and *Raynaud's phenomenon.* All of these features, particularly Raynaud's phenomenon (which is what happens when your fingers become patriotic by turning red, white, and blue when exposed to cold temperatures), are prominent features of autoimmune diseases such as systemic lupus erythematosus and seleroderma, which are also characterized by dysautonomia and neurogenic inflammation. We have seen patients erroneously diagnosed with lupus who really had fibromyalgia with dysautonomia.

Fibromyalgia and Dysautonomia

Abnormal autonomic regulation leads to many secondary clinical syndromes that can be part of fibromyalgia or fall into the realm of *fibromyalgia-associated conditions.* Most of these conditions are discussed in detail later and are listed in Table 5. They include mitral valve prolapse, noncardiac chest pain, migraine/tension headaches, irritable bowel syndrome (also called *spastic colitis* or *functional bowel syndrome*), premenstrual syndrome, and irritable bladder.

Infrequently, serious derangements of the ANS lead to prolonged stimulation of pain amplifiers, which results in chronic neurogenic inflammation. The most important complication of this is a condition of sympathetically mediated pain known as *reflex sympathetic dystrophy.*

Table 5. *Examples of autonomic dysfunction in fibromyalgia*

Neurally mediated hypotension—abnormally low blood pressure

Mitral valve prolapse—causes palpitations due to release of epinephrine, which increases heart rates

Neurogenic inflammation—swelling on an autonomic basis

Reflex sympathetic dystrophy—neurogenic inflammation with severe pain

Migraine headaches—autonomically mediated abnormal dilation of brain blood vessels

Numbness, tingling, burning—when abnormal vascular tone or neurogenic inflammation presses on nerves or activates their sensors

Livedo reticularis and palmar erythema—loss of autonomic control in capillaries under the skin and increased flow through small, superficial arteries

Cognitive dysfunction—autonomically mediated abnormal constriction of brain blood vessels

It has been postulated that a hypervigilance is associated with dysautonomia that results in fibromyalgia patients becoming acutely aware of normal bodily activities. Patients report being uncomfortable as they feel palpitations or experience spasm in the abdomen, or have difficulty tolerating daily noises.

The Autonomic Nervous System: Summing Up

Regulation of autonomic control may be abnormal in fibromyalgia. Autonomic dysregulation can mimic some features observed in autoimmune disease and is often mistaken for them. Many commonly observed complaints in fibromyalgia, such as irritable colon, mitral valve prolapse, edema, reddish discoloration of the skin, and tension headaches, are due in part to abnormalities of the ANS.

4
Fibromyalgia-Related Complaints

Fibromyalgia is a syndrome rather than a disease, and as such has a variety of features. Any part of the body can be involved, especially when fibromyalgia is induced or aggravated by multiple factors.

CONSTITUTIONAL SYMPTOMS AND SIGNS

Complaints can be subjective and hard to verify or quantify. They consist of *symptoms,* or expressions of what is bothersome, and *signs.* Physical signs are observed during a physical examination, such as a rash or an irregular heartbeat, and are easier to validate. Constitutional symptoms or signs are generalized and do not belong to any specific organ system or region of the body.

Fatigue

Generalized fatigue is a prominent feature of fibromyalgia. Between 60 and 80 percent of fibromyalgia patients complain of *fatigue,* which is defined as physical or mental exhaustion or weariness. However, there are many reasons for fatigue. In a recent survey, 20 percent of the women in the United States and 14 percent of the men rated themselves as being significantly fatigued. This feeling can come on like a wave or be continuous. Some of the basic causes of fatigue include emotional stress, depression, physical illness, poor sleeping, and poor eating. Examples of fatigue-inducing conditions include working too hard, substance abuse, anemia, low thyroid level, side effects of medication, overtraining, menopause, pregnancy, diabetes, heart disease, kidney impairment, cancer, depression, excessive perfectionist tendencies, autoimmune disease, and inflammation. The majority of patients with fibromyalgia and chronic, otherwise unexplained fatigue in whom a primary psychiatric diagnosis has been ruled out also meet the criteria for chronic fatigue syndrome.

Do Fibromyalgia Patients Run Fevers?

Everybody has a temperature, but few people run persistent fevers. A *fever* is defined as a body temperature above 99.6° F. Occasionally, patients complain to their doctor about recurrent fevers and relate that their baseline temperatures are usually 96–97° F. Therefore, the normal temperature obtained at examination is a fever. Twenty percent of fibromyalgia patients include fevers in their list of complaints. Many, in fact, feel feverish. Hot and cold sweats or the sensation of "burning up" are not uncommon in fibromyalgia patients and reflect dysautonomia. Thirty percent with fibromyalgia relate some degree of cold intolerance. Verifiable, chronic fever is *not* a feature of primary fibromyalgia but an indication that another condition is causing fibromyalgia-like complaints. Inflammatory conditions, infections, and tumors should be sought out.

Swollen or Tender Glands

The body's lymphatic system is a network of glands or lymph nodes that assist veins in clearing up water and debris and returning fluid from the arms, legs, and other areas of the body to the heart area. An infection such as a sore throat can lead to swollen lymph nodes in the neck area. Chronic poor circulation can produce edema from poor lymph drainage or varicose veins in the legs. Most lymph glands are enlarged when we have a local infection, an inflammation, or a malignancy.

Twenty percent of fibromyalgia patients complain of having swollen lymph nodes. Many who have a postinfectious fatigue syndrome start out with swollen glands, but the glands are no longer enlarged by the time a fibromyalgia specialist is consulted. Those who are thin also have relatively prominent lymph nodes, a condition not associated with any disease. As with a fever, if the doctor can feel the lymph nodes in a given area, this is not due to fibromyalgia but represents a circulation problem, allergic reaction, infection, inflammatory process, cancer, or simply bodily thinness.

The perception of tender lymph glands is common in fibromyalgia and reflects allodynia. The glands themselves are not enlarged or abnormal under the microscope.

FIBROMYALGIA IN MEN

Since 90 percent with fibromyalgia are females, does the syndrome differ in males? Men with fibromyalgia tend to have more severe symptoms, poorer physical functioning, and a lower quality of life. Hormones probably play a role in pain perception. It has been suggested that healthy males make 40 percent less serotonin than healthy women. We are not quite sure what this means, but even though women have lower tender point pain thresholds, men complain of "hurting all over" more often.

MUSCLE FINDINGS: WEAKNESS, MYALGIAS, LACK OF ENDURANCE, AND SPASM

Over 80 percent of fibromyalgia patients have muscular symptoms or signs. Aching in the muscles, or *myalgias,* is common in the upper or lower back and neck areas. Myalgias are usually present on both the right and left sides and present as a dull, throbbing discomfort. *Spasm,* defined as an involuntary muscular contraction, is less common than the sense of tightness in muscles that seems like spasm. Muscular aches tend to worsen after exercise and activity and as the day wears on. The discomfort is generally more severe in the late afternoons and feels "flu-like."

What is going on in the muscles? As discussed earlier, the muscles are weak only if deconditioning is present. Areas of taut bands may be felt as tender points. Some fibromyalgia patients who once engaged in vigorous exercise complain that they feel exhausted after a short workout and no longer have endurance. How does this happen? Postexertional pain occurs when arteries in the muscle constrict and not enough oxygen gets to these areas. Exercise requires increased oxygen to the muscles, and the lack of oxygen produces muscle pain. Fibromyalgia patients don't use oxygen optimally and prematurely deplete their energy reserves. This leads to deconditioning and produces a vicious cycle that promotes a fear of exercise.

Myalgias should be differentiated from inflammation of the muscles, which is known as *myositis,* and other conditions associated with aching muscles. Inflammatory processes such as polymyositis or systemic lupus can mimic fibromyalgia, as can a low thyroid blood level, my-asthenia gravis, multiple sclerosis, infections, and anemia. Common prescription medications (e.g., "statin" cholesterol drugs, colchicine) infrequently induce side effects affecting muscles, which leads to aching or weakness. Inflammatory myositis, hypothyroidism, and the above-mentioned drugs can produce abnormally high blood levels of the muscle enzyme creatine phosphokinase (CPK) or abnormal electrical tracings in muscles on an electromyogram (EMG).

SOFT TISSUE AND JOINT COMPLAINTS: WIDESPREAD PAIN, ARTHRALGIAS, AND STIFFNESS

The International Association for the Study of Pain has defined *pain* as an unpleasant sensory and emotional experience. Widespread pain (from pain amplification) is such a prominent feature of fibromyalgia syndrome that it is included in the definition of the syndrome. The pain usually emanates from the soft tissues, muscles, and joints. Soft tissues include the supporting structures of joints such as tendons, bursae, and ligaments, as well as the myofascia. The myofascia lies between the lower skin (dermis) and muscles and consists of connective tissue and fat, which buffer muscles and provide structural integrity and support. The nature of the pain is highly variable. Some patients use descriptive terms such as *aching, burning, gnawing, smarting,* or *throbbing.* Pain can change sites and often gets better or worse on its own. Tender points are common in myofascial planes.

Fibromyalgia does not damage or inflame joints, but it can produce joint complaints. More than 80 percent of patients with fibromyalgia describe symptoms of aching in their joints, or *arthralgias,* and 60 percent have stiffness. Many patients also have other forms of arthritis, especially osteoarthritis, and a few have autoimmune disorders such as lupus or rheumatoid arthritis with a secondary fibromyalgia.

Whereas morning stiffness is an important feature of osteoarthritis and rheumatoid arthritis, most fibromyalgia patients become stiff in the late afternoon and early evening or when they have been in one position for a prolonged period of time. Stiffness is a difficult sensation to convey to others. Rheumatologists use the term *gelling* to denote the jello-like feeling of the stiff, tightened joints, muscles, and soft tissues of fibromyalgia. It improves when you move around, apply heat, or take a hot shower.

MUSCULAR CONTRACTION (TENSION) AND MIGRAINE HEADACHES

Most fibromyalgia patients complain of recurrent headaches. These headaches usually are one of two types: tension or migraine. Tension headaches are muscular contraction headaches. Patients describe these headaches as a dull "tight band around the head" similar to what they feel in other muscles of the body. A sustained muscle contraction can compress small vessels in the area. Tension headaches frequently involve the forehead, jaw, and temple areas. Occipital headaches, or pain in the upper part of the back of the neck, can be a type of tension headache and are associated with muscle spasm or stiffness. Osteoarthritis of the cervical spine can also cause occipital headaches. On occasion, moving the neck in any direction is painful. Tension headaches usually respond to the same remedies used to treat myalgias, arthralgias, and spasm.

Ten percent of the U.S. population suffers from vascular-mediated migraine headaches. Usually one-sided, associated with light sensitivity (photophobia), manifested by pounding, and preceded by a premonition of coming on, migraines occur in 20 percent of patients with fibromyalgia. Low serotonin levels are found in migraine sufferers, which in turn can alter vascular tone. Physiologically, a migraine begins with constriction of blood vessels (which produces the premonition, or aura) followed by dilatation. When arteries dilate, the stretching of the blood vessel and nerves evokes an intense headache.

Migraines are much more common in fibromyalgia patients who have ANS dysfunction. They complain of a throbbing or aching on one side of the head. This can be coupled with nausea or vomiting, visual disturbance (ocular migraine), or dizziness. Migraines can be brought on by unpleasant emotional stress, certain foods, menstruation, weather changes, smoke, hunger, or fatigue.

SLEEP ABNORMALITIES: NONRESTORATIVE SLEEP, SLEEP MYOCLONUS, BRUXISM

Sleep is necessary to promote the production of chemicals important in tissue growth and maintenance of immune function. As was mentioned in Chapter 3, nonrestorative (or nonrefreshing) sleep is found in most fibromyalgia patients. We all go through four stages of sleep, ranging from light to deep, where brain waves are denoted by the Greek letters alpha, beta, gamma, and delta. Persistent alpha wave intrusion into slow delta wave sleep results in waking up feeling sore all over and sometimes feeling more tired than when going to bed. Fibromyalgia patients make less growth hormone (which has little to do with growing in adults but is essential to maintain certain body functions) than healthy people while asleep, which can accelerate muscle injury and increase pain levels. These electrical abnormalities can be documented with a brain wave sleep study, known as a polysomnogram or a sleep electroencephalogram.

Ten percent of patients with fibromyalgia also suffer from a poorly understood condition known as *sleep myoclonus*; their legs suddenly shoot out, lift, jerk, or go into spasm. Sometimes called *restless legs syndrome,* or periodic limb movement syndrome (PMLS) which also can occur when awake, this condition reflects a lack of oxygen in muscles and other tissues in the legs and is not unique to fibromyalgia. Additionally, some fibromyalgia patients grind their teeth when they sleep. Known as *bruxism,* this represents a tightening of the jaw muscles.

COGNITIVE IMPAIRMENT, OR "BRAIN FATIGUE"

Some of our fibromyalgia patients are concerned because they cannot think clearly, remember names and dates, balance their checkbooks, or add numbers the way they once did. Characterized by confusion, memory blanks, word mix-ups, and concentration difficulties, these changes are often subtle and imperceptible to the physician who hears the complaint. Cognitive impairment, which some patients term *brain fatigue* or *fibrofog*, is found in 20 percent of fibromyalgia patients. These complaints may be fleeting, intermittent, or constant and until recently were attributed to depression or stress. Additionally, some patients describe dizziness (which is not movement related), clumsiness and dropping things (which are not part of neurologic diseases such as multiple sclerosis), or visual changes or eye pain (which are not part of migraines). If these concerns are not handled wisely, patients are more likely to secondarily develop anxiety, panic, mood swings, and irritability.

For years, rheumatologists were as guilty as other doctors of ascribing cognitive impairment to depression or stress. How else could they explain the normal findings on neurologic examinations, MRI scans of the brain, and spinal fluid tests? However, on the basis of recently published work, we now know that cognitive impairment is real, and we are working hard to educate our colleagues.

Two lines of evidence provide support for the concept of non-psychological cognitive dysfunction. First, in Chapter 3 we discussed the role of cytokines, chemicals that induce cognitive impairment along with fibromyalgia. Evidence suggests that cytokine function is abnormally regulated. Second, by employing the SPECT imaging technique, Dr. Larry Bradley and his colleagues at the University of Alabama have convincingly shown that fibromyalgia patients do not get enough oxygen to specific parts of their brains on an intermittent basis. Looking at the problem from a different angle, ANS abnormalities occasionally may produce enough spasm in cerebral blood vessels to deprive regions of the brain of oxygen. Interestingly, nonrestorative sleep by itself can produce these SPECT scanning abnormalities.

Serious, obvious cognitive dysfunction is uncommon, found in less than 5 percent of fibromyalgia patients.

NUMBNESS, BURNING, AND TINGLING

At some time, one-third of fibromyalgia patients will become aware of a vague sensation of numbness, tingling, or burning. These symptoms may be reported in any part of the body and tend to come and go. When neurologists are consulted, their physical findings are usually within normal limits. Muscle and nerve blood tests are also normal. Although diagnostic electrical evaluations with an EMG or a nerve conduction study can identify cervical or lumbar disc problems, diabetes or other metabolic abnormalities, inflammation, or compressive lesions such as carpal tunnel syndrome, these studies are normal in primary fibromyalgia.

Carpal tunnel syndrome consists of compression of the median nerve at the wrist as it enters the palm of the hand. Its prevalence is increased among fibromyalgia patients, especially those who work with computers all day and others with poor workstation body mechanics. Carpal tunnel syndrome is usually treated by splinting, local steroid injections, and, if needed, an occupational or physical therapy evaluation. Anybody suspected of having carpal tunnel syndrome should have a confirmatory median sensory nerve conduction study of the upper extremity before undergoing corrective surgery. Since hand numbness is a feature of *both* fibromyalgia and carpal tunnel syndrome, some patients have had expensive and unnecessary surgery that fails to relieve the numbness and tingling of fibromyalgia. Unfortunately, we have observed the distinctive scar on the inside surface of the wrist indicating carpal tunnel surgery in about 10 percent of our patients, many of whom did not require surgery.

Why should numbness and tingling be a feature of fibromyalgia? Painful nerve sensations are a mild form of neurogenic inflammation or local nerve compression caused by autonomic dysfunction. Unless reflex sympathetic dystrophy is present, it should evoke little concern. Although annoying and a cause of aggravated poor sleep, fibromyalgia neuralgia (painful nerve symptoms) never causes paralysis, strokes, or deformity.

DRY EYES AND OTHER EYE OR EAR COMPLAINTS

Dry eyes or dry mouth, also known as *sicca symptoms,* have been reported in 10–35 percent of fibromyalgia patients. Manifested by burning, stinging, and redness of the eyes and verified by pits in the cornea on a Rose Bengal stain, diminished tearing in fibromyalgia has been attributed to altered autonomic nervous system activity. These small, difficult-to-see pits occur when the cornea does not receive enough moisture. Dry eyes are much more common than dry mouth.

Sicca related to fibromyalgia should be differentiated from an autoimmune-mediated dry eyes, dry mouth, and arthritis condition known as *Sjogren's syndrome,* in which autoantibodies are usually present. In Sjogren's syndrome, viral infections (as in AIDS or the mumps), alcoholism, and metabolic illnesses, the parotid (salivary) gland within the cheeks may become enlarged. Since tricyclic antidepressants are one of the principal treatments for fibromyalgia, and frequently cause dry eyes and dry mouth, it is sometimes difficult to ascertain how many people truly have fibromyalgia syndrome-induced dryness syndrome.

WHY AM I DIZZY? WHY DO NORMAL NOISES BOTHER ME?

More patients with fibromyalgia complain of feeling dizzy than otherwise healthy people. Dizziness can be a result of a bone spur in the neck causing pressure on the blood supply of the brain, chronic allergies with sinus inflammation, migraine, low blood pressure, medications, palpitations from autonomically mediated mitral valve prolapse, or a thyroid imbalance. Some fibromyalgia patients without these problems also notice a sensation of dizziness. Studies have suggested that the vestibular, or equilibrium, center in the ears is not optimally regulated in fibromyalgia patients. The reason is not well understood, but it may have to do with autonomic lack of blood flow to the vestibular center. Some fibromyalgia patients may have a low frequency nerve-mediated hearing loss that is asymptomatic. Recent evidence suggests that these fibromyalgia patients are not really dizzy. Dizziness is a sensation of being in motion, but what some fibromyalgia patients are experiencing is *vertigo,* a malfunction of the vestibular center of the ear producing a sensation that everything around you is in motion. Some fibromyalgia patients have decreased noise tolerance on the basis of a hypervigilant vestibular reaction. Chemicals can also elicit stimuli that sensitize the limbic system (Chapter 3) through "limbic kindling" that facilitates behavioral, autonomic, hormonal, and immune functions, producing "dizziness." Additionally, some fibromyalgia therapies, such as nonsteroidal anti-inflammatory drugs (NSAIDs), can lead to complaints of ringing in the ears, or *tinnitus,* or rarely, in other patients, diminished hearing.

CHEST COMPLAINTS: PALPITATIONS, COSTOCHONDRITIS, AND NONCARDIAC CHEST PAIN

Although some patients are concerned that their critical organs are involved in fibromyalgia, chest area symptoms infrequently are related to heart or lung disease. Palpitations, noncardiac chest pain, and subjective swelling or edema are important symptoms and signs of fibromyalgia. Reflux from the esophagus, gastrointestinal complaints, and female organ-related problems are also reviewed in this chapter in the context of fibromyalgia-associated concerns.

The sense of having extra heartbeats, or *palpitations,* is reported in 10–20 percent of patients with fibromyalgia. Although heart disease, caffeine intake, anxiety, and other factors are associated with palpitations, many otherwise healthy young women have *mitral valve prolapse.* The prevalence of mitral valve prolapse is clearly increased in fibromyalgia. The mitral valve, one of the four valves of the heart that lies between its right-sided chambers, can become more floppy under ANS influence and produce palpitations. Patients feel as though they will pass out but rarely do. Mitral valve prolapse is also associated with chest pains and shortness of breath and can be easily diagnosed by a heart ultrasound known as a *two-dimensional echocardiogram.* Most patients with mitral valve prolapse do not require medication, and benefit from avoiding caffeine and learning how to relax. However, between 5–10 percent of these patients are referred to a cardiologist because they have potentially serious heart irregularities and may benefit from the initiation of heart drugs known as *beta blockers.*

There is no question that costochondritis can be scary. The sternum, or breast bone, is connected to ribs by a rope-like tethering tissue. When this tissue (known as the *costochondral margin)* becomes irritated, it causes discomfort, especially in smokers, persons with lung disease or large breasts, and persons with inflammatory disorders such as rheumatoid arthritis. As noted in Figures 1 and 7, the costochondral margins are two of the tender points found in fibromyalgia. Sometimes referred to as *Tietze's syndrome,* this irritation produces chest pains. It sometimes takes an emergency room visit by a patient who is concerned about possibly having a heart attack before fibromyalgia is ultimately diagnosed. Costochondritis can be differentiated from cardiac pain because even though the sternum-rib attachments are tender to the touch, palpating the center of the sternum does not produce pain. A doctor may order chest or rib X-rays to make sure that there is no fracture.

Sometimes, patients with fibromyalgia report that it hurts when they take a deep breath. They fear it might be *pleurisy,* or irritation of the lining of the lung, which is extremely common in autoimmune diseases. Another form of noncardiac chest pain relates to spasm of the *esophagus.*

DOCTOR, CAN'T YOU SEE HOW SWOLLEN I AM?

One area of conflict we have observed between doctors and fibromyalgia patients involves the physician's skepticism that a fluid retention problem is really present. Women with fibromyalgia frequently

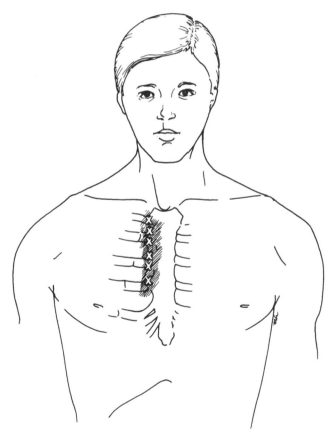

Fig. 7 *Costochondritis. The Xs mark potentially painful areas where ribs attach to the sternum.*

report fluid retention and swelling. However, physical examinations and routine testing usually fail to document objective swelling. When doctors respond instinctively and prescribe a diuretic, or water pill, the fibromyalgia worsens because these preparations mobilize fluid by promoting muscle actions that induce more pain. Too many of these patients unfortunately become dependent on diuretics and gain 5–10 pounds within days when a different doctor or the patient stops the drug. Tricyclics in higher doses, particularly doxepin (Sinequan), can cause fluid retention as well.

Research from Great Britain has suggested that there is subclinical swelling, or fluid retention that is not noticeable on classic palpation, an electrocardiogram, chest X-ray, or pitting on physical examination. These studies provide evidence that in fibromyalgia autonomically mediated sympathetic nervous system hypofunction induces neurogenic vasodilatation (see Chapter 3). This leads to decreased arterial vessel tone, which produces decreased capillary flow and results in increased capillary leakage of sodium and water. The net result is a perceived loss of volume by the kidney, which reflexively secretes chemicals that promote salt and water retention, or edema. Premenstrual acceleration of this phenomenon is common.

SKIN COMPLAINTS

Some fibromyalgia patients have more than tender points under their skin. The skin itself is tender to touch. A manifestation of widespread allodynia, or heightened pain perception, this discomfort is present in more severe cases and is especially prevalent in patients taking steroids and in those who develop reflex sympathetic dystrophy. There is no rash, per se, that is a unique feature of fibromyalgia. More patients than would be expected in the general population report dry skin, hair loss, itching, mouth sores, and easy bruisibility, although none of these complaints has yet been studied scientifically to determine if specific dermatologic problems are associated with fibromyalgia. Fibromyalgia patients also take more aspirin, ibuprofen, and other NSAIDs, which can result in black-and-blue marks under the skin.

As discussed earlier, autonomic dysfunction produces changes under the skin that mimic Raynaud's phenomenon and cause livedo reticularis, the lace-like mottling of the skin that usually produces no symptoms (see Chapter 4). It's not uncommon for fibromyalgia patients to have a ruddy complexion or red palms along with this condition.

Gastrointestinal and genitourinary complaints are reviewed in Chapter 6.

SUMMING UP

A surprisingly wide range of multisystemic symptoms and signs in healthy-appearing people can be a source of frustration and misunderstanding among patients, family members, and physicians. Many of these complaints are part of regional fibromyalgia syndromes, or *fibromyalgia-associated conditions,* which are reviewed in the next three chapters. Table 6 lists the frequency of the principal complaints among fibromyalgia patients.

Table 6. *Prevalence (%) of frequently observed symptoms and signs in fibromyalgia*

Widespread pain with tender points	100
Generalized weakness, muscle and joint aches	80
Unrefreshing sleep	80
Fatigue	70
Stiffness	60
Tension headache	53
Painful periods	40
Irritable colon, functional bowel disease	40
Subjective numbness, swelling, tingling	35
Skin redness, lace-like red skin mottling	30
Complaints of fever	20
Complaints of swollen glands	20
Complaints of dry eyes	20
Subjective significant cognitive dysfunction	20
Significant psychopathology	5–20
Nocturnal myoclonus, restless legs syndrome	15
Female urethral syndrome, irritable bladder	12
Vulvodynia or vaginismus	10
Concomitant reflex sympathetic dystrophy	5

5

What Are the Regional and Localized Forms of Fibromyalgia?

The definition of fibromyalgia includes widespread pain in all four quadrants (areas) of the body. What happens when you have fibromyalgia-like pain located in only one or two quadrants of the body? Limited forms of the syndrome have distinct features and terms used to describe them. *Myofascial pain syndrome* encompasses many regional pain conditions ranging from temporomandibular joint dysfunction in the jaw to a low back pain syndrome. The diagnosis of myofascial pain syndrome requires that at least one trigger point be present and that, when it is pressed, pain is referred to another site. This chapter will review regional myofascial pain, relate it to fibromyalgia pain pathways, and discuss its management and prognosis.

WHAT CAUSES REGIONAL MYOFASCIAL PAIN?

Most regional myofascial discomfort is produced by trauma. Unlike fibromyalgia, in which nearly 50 inciting factors have been implicated, localized or regional myofascial pain syndrome is usually due to either a single traumatic event or repetitive injury.

Numerous factors contribute to myofascial problems. The term *myofascia* refers to both muscles (myo-) and the *fascia*, the thin layer of tissue covering, supporting, and separating muscles. Abnormal posture can produce local discomfort. For example, scoliosis may be associated with midback or scapular pain on one side. A patient who has had lower extremity orthopedic surgery and needs to walk with a cane or crutch for a few weeks and is not used to it may place abnormal stress on the back, hips, shoulder, or elbow, resulting in a temporary regional pain syndrome.

From a physiologic standpoint, most of the neurochemical pathways reviewed in Chapter 3 play a role in regional body syndromes. However, in regional myofascial pain, more emphasis is placed on sensitization of a primary nociceptor, a nerve that receives painful stimuli and transmits that information to the spinal cord. This results in secondary hyperalgesia (more pain than would normally be expected in an area), allodynia (an ordinarily painless stimulus that produces pain), and/or referred pain. Pain that occurs from stretching a muscle is due to a reflex spasm secondary to altered peripheral nociception elsewhere. Prolonged shortening of a muscle increases pain, as does overuse in the form of a sustained muscle contraction.

Tender points play a major role in regional musculoskeletal pain. Tender points are hyperirritable loci found at muscle-tendon junctions near nerves where mechanical forces cause microinjuries. Researchers have found vasoconstriction in the skin above, along with a slightly lower temperature, indicating that the ANS plays a role here. Local injury of tender points decreases the firing threshold of nerves as the stimulation of local nociceptors promotes the release of cytokines. *Referred pain* relates to discomfort in areas that are near but not in the injured region or the affected tender points. Referred pain is produced by altered central nociception and enlarged receptor fields. Nociceptor input can be referred to another area served by receptors that converge in the spinothalamic tract. It can be very misleading. For instance, suppose that an area on the left side near your midcervical spine is extremely uncomfortable. The traumatic insult that led to this condition might be in the back of the shoulder, but pain is referred to this area near the spine. For therapists, focusing rehabilitation energies on areas of referred pain is not as rewarding as dealing with the primary, inciting biochemical problem. Figures 8–10 illustrate examples of referred pain.

WHAT DOES A DOCTOR EXPECT TO SEE IN REGIONAL FORMS OF FIBROMYALGIA?

Patients with regional myofascial pain syndrome generally do not fulfill the ACR criteria for fibromyalgia. A distinct minority of patients with regional myofascial pain have systemic symptoms associated with fibromyalgia, such as fatigue, poor concentration, bloating, generalized weakness, and nonrestorative sleep. They tend to be slightly younger than most fibromyalgia patients and include more males. Pain occurs in an injured area long beyond its expected normal healing time and is chronic due to altered nociception or abnormal transmission of pain signals.

Myofascial pain syndrome can occur anywhere in the body, but more than 90 percent of these cases involve one of the following five

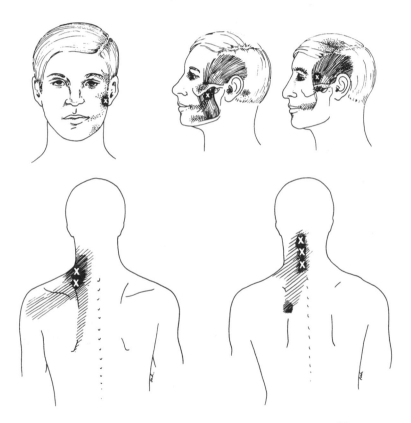

Fig. 8 *(top) TMJ dysfunction syndrome: tender points (X) and referred pain areas.*
Fig. 9 *(bottom left) Upper back (trapezius) tender points (X) and areas of referred pain.*
Fig. 10 *(bottom right) Occipital (back of the neck) tender points (X) and referred pain areas.*

regional combinations: neck and upper torso; temporomandibular joint (atypical facial pain, or TMJ); neck, arm, hand; low back, buttock, leg; and the chest area, including costochondritis. See Figures 8–10 for examples.

EXAMPLES OF WELL-KNOWN SUBSETS OF REGIONAL MYOFASCIAL PAIN

Two of the best-known examples of regional myofascial pain involve jaw discomfort and repetitive strain disorder. Most TMJ patients consult ear, nose, or throat specialists, dentists, or orthopedists, as opposed to rheumatologists. In more serious cases, localized symptoms ultimately are connected to a systemic process such as fibromyalgia.

TMJ Dysfunction Syndrome

Jaw pain is very uncomfortable and stems from many different sources. These include malocclusion, or an abnormal bite; arthritis of the joint (in rheumatoid arthritis and, to a less severe degree, in osteoarthritis); infection; bruxism, or teeth grinding; and traumatic injury. Myofascial pain from muscular spasm, with or without upper back and neck pain on the affected side, is a diagnosis of exclusion termed *temporomandibular joint dysfunction syndrome*. The pain stems from the same sources causing fibromyalgia and is amplified by anxiety, stress, or trauma, leading to unconscious jaw-closing movements. This regional form of fibromyalgia is diagnosed only after a dental evaluation and an ear, nose, and throat evaluation by a specialist, along with a special type of X-ray or imaging scan of the TMJ.

TMJ dysfunction syndrome afflicts 10 million Americans; 70 percent are female. In a recent survey, 18 percent fulfilled the criteria for fibromyalgia and 75 percent of those with fibromyalgia had TMJ dysfunction. The temples, neck, and upper back can be affected. The TMJ dysfunction syndrome is treated with NSAIDs such as ibuprofen or naproxen, as well as moist heat, joint spacers (bite plates) worn at night, exercises, and a technique known as *spray and stretch*. Occasionally, injecting the TMJ joint with a small amount of steroid and a local anesthetic such as xylocaine may be useful. Most general management features that are reviewed later may also be recommended or prescribed. Once the diagnosis of TMJ syndrome is made, expensive and unnecessary surgery should be avoided except in extreme cases and only after several expert opinions are obtained.

Repetitive Strain Syndrome

Over the last few years, Geoffrey Littlejohn and his associates in Australia have performed pioneering work on musculoskeletal problems observed in the workplace. With Australia's generous worker's compensation system and excellent data collection methodologies, his group helped nurture our current concepts of repetitive stress syndromes. A discipline known as *ergonomics,* which is a hybrid of kinesiology (the science or study of movement), engineering, and physics, has explored the science of human performance at work. Practitioners have developed information about what types of local stress individuals can sustain in a work environment over a period of time. For example, working at a computer all day or lifting shipping cartons onto a truck are forms of repetitive strain. Many patients in the former category might complain of pain in the shoulder, with numbness and tingling in the hand. Anti-inflammatory medication, physical therapy, and even a local injection of an anesthetic, with or without corticosteroids, is only temporarily beneficial if the fundamental ergonomics of the workstation are not adapted to the patient's requirements. Some of these considerations, along with disability issues, are reviewed in more detail in Chapter 11.

If repetitive strain syndrome is not adequately addressed and the patient continues to engage in an ergonomically unsatisfactory job environment, not only might disability and chronic regional pain be the consequence, but full-blown fibromyalgia can evolve.

WHAT'S THE PROGNOSIS?

The outcome of regional pain syndromes is generally very good to excellent, usually much better than that of fibromyalgia. Delays in treatment, incorrect treatment, or continued injury to the effected region have adverse consequences that can allow fibromyalgia to develop.

6

What Conditions Are Associated with Fibromyalgia?

Throughout this century, patients with fibromyalgia-like complaints have been diagnosed by physicians as having all types of conditions, syndromes, and diseases. Many of these overlap with fibromyalgia, and this chapter focuses on the most important ones.

CHRONIC FATIGUE SYNDROME

The codification and "legitimization" of fibromyalgia with statistically validated criteria has paralleled similar initiatives concerning chronic fatigue syndrome (CFS). Chapter 1 recounted some of the earlier insights and efforts. An acute infection is often characterized by fever, swollen glands, and either a cold/bronchitis, a stomach/intestinal condition, or an aching/debilitating presentation. As the body fights infection and makes antibodies against microbes, acute symptoms and signs start to disappear and most of the time patients feel much better. However, a variety of organisms can stimulate the production of cytokines (discussed in Chapter 3) and other chemicals, which prolong fatigue and aching and may be associated with cognitive impairment, malaise, pain amplification, and sleeping difficulties.

How the Centers for Disease Control
Drew Up Criteria for CFS

Between 1930 and 1980, it was known that some patients recovering from infectious diseases such as polio, mononucleosis, and brucellosis had a prolonged convalescence and persistent systemic symptoms. By the early 1980s, a herpesvirus known as Epstein-Barr virus joined the group (mononucleosis is also a herpesvirus). For unknown reasons, it tended to afflict upwardly mobile young people, and the press tagged Epstein-Barr virus as a "yuppie flu disease." Epstein-Barr virus antibodies could easily be tested for, and its postviral fatigue complaints were treated symptomatically and waited out.

However, the "Epstein-Barr syndrome" epidemic turned out not to happen. The National Institutes of Health, United States Centers for Disease Control and Prevention (CDC), and other centers showed that over half of the U.S. population has evidence of exposure to Epstein-Barr virus in their blood, and standard antiviral therapy for herpes was not beneficial in these patients. The CDC devised statistically validated criteria for CFS in 1988, which were updated in 1994 (Table 7). The current definition of CFS requires unexplained, clinically evaluated fatigue of new or definite onset lasting for at least six months and not relieved with rest that substantially impairs performance. New onset of four of the following eight factors must also be present: cognitive impairment, sore throat, tender cervical or axillary lymph nodes, muscle aches, joint aches, headache, sleep disorder, and malaise after exertion lasting longer than one day. By definition, patients with primary psychiatric disorders cannot have CFS. Using the aforementioned criteria, the prevalence of CFS in the United States is somewhere between 100,000 and 300,000, with several hundred thousand other persons having unexplained chronic fatigue without CFS. According to a study conducted in Great Britain, 4 percent of the population complained of

Table 7. *The CDC revised criteria for CFS (1994)*

1. Chronic fatigue of unknown cause that persists or returns for more than 6 months, resulting in a substantial reduction in occupational, educational, social, or personal activities.
2. The presence of 4 or more of the following symptoms concurrently for more than 6 months:
   a. Sore throat
   b. Tender cervical or axillary lymph glands
   c. Muscle pain
   d. Multijoint pain
   e. New headaches
   f. Unrefreshing sleep
   g. Postexertion malaise
   h. Cognitive dysfunction

chronic fatigue. If coexisting psychiatric and medical disorders were excluded, 0.5 percent of the population fulfilled criteria for CFS.

Sometimes, CFS is referred to as *chronic fatigue immune dysfunction syndrome (CFIDS)*. The authors prefer the term *CFS* since immune dysfunction is neither a proven nor prominent feature of the syndrome.

CFS and Fibromyalgia: Similarities and Differences

The majority of patients diagnosed with CFS in the United States are between the ages of 20 and 50, female, and Caucasian. Comparative surveys show that 20–70 percent of fibromyalgia patients have CFS, and 35–70 percent of those with CFS have fibromyalgia. CFS patients have greater elevations of antiviral antibodies than is observed in fibromyalgia. Whereas only a minority of fibromyalgia patients complain of a sore throat, show evidence of swollen glands or fevers, and have onset after a flu-like illness, these features are found in most CFS patients (Table 8). Although one well-regarded theory suggests that CFS is manifested after exposure to repeated viral infections in the setting of an overactive immune state, immune blood testing is inconsistent, contradictory, expensive, and does not change our treatment.

Table 8. *Comparisons of fibromyalgia and CFS*

Parameter	Fibromyalgia (%)	Chronic fatigue syndrome (%)
Female sex	90	80
Muscle aches	99	80
Joint aches	99	75
Fatigue	90	99
Poor sleep	80	50
Complaints of fever	28	75
Complaints of swollen glands	33	80
Postexertional fatigue	80	80
Sudden or acute onset	55	70
Headaches	60	85
Cognitive dysfunction	20	65

Autonomic dysfunction is common in CFS. This leads to low blood pressure in many of these patients, which is manifested clinically as *neurally mediated hypotension* that aggravates fatigue. Here sympathetic activity produces a low resting volume. This excessive pooling of blood on dependent vessels produces an excessive loss of plasma when standing up. Cognitive impairment has also been documented with hypoperfusion on SPECT scanning, with the brain intermittently not getting enough oxygen.

THE FUNCTIONAL BOWEL SPECTRUM

Over the last decade, functional bowel disease has become a spectrum of gastroenterologic disorders with a common link of *visceral hyperalgesia,* or increased pain sensitivity in the internal structures. Identified by a variety of terms including *spastic colitis, irritable colon, diffuse abdominal pain, noncardiac chest pain,* and *nonulcer dyspepsia,* this spectrum was once primarily thought to be a motility, or movement, disorder. In fact, it has turned out to be a pain amplification disorder. Initiated by inciting factors that cause peripheral or visceral pain fibers and the parasympathetic nervous system to promote primary and secondary hyperalgesia with central sensitization, the functional bowel spectrum substantially overlaps with fibromyalgia. Patients report increased perception of stomach movements and distension. This lower sensory threshold leads to abdominal pain and discomfort.

Functional bowel complaints are the most common reason for referral to a gastroenterologist. As with fibromyalgia, 2 percent of the U.S. population fulfill the criteria for functional bowel disease, but as many as 20 percent may have it at some point. In the United States, 70 percent are female, and it costs $8 billion a year to diagnose and treat it. Patients report abdominal distention, bloating, pain relief with bowel movements, more frequent and loose stools with the onset of pain, frequent mucus in bowel movements, a sensation of incomplete evacuation, flatulence, and cramping. Some doctors believe that food allergies or medication sensitivity aggravate the syndrome.

Fibromyalgia complaints extend beyond the small intestine or colon. For example, sensitization of different parts of the spinal cord and referred pain can lead to persistent upper abdominal nonulcer pain and chest pains. Recent studies suggest that approximately 40 percent of patients with functional bowel disease fulfill the criteria for fibromyalgia and vice versa. Functional bowel disease affects a type of muscle known as *involuntary,* or *smooth,* muscle. By contrast, fibromyalgia tender points overlie voluntary, striated, or skeletal muscle.

AUTOIMMUNE DISEASES

Autoimmune rheumatic diseases are inflammatory processes in which the body makes antibodies to its own tissues, in essence becoming allergic to itself. On occasion, it may be difficult to differentiate these conditions from fibromyalgia. Untreated inflammation associated with autoimmunity may induce a secondary fibromyalgia, as might changing the doses of corticosteroids used to treat it. Surveys suggest that 7 percent of patients with Sjogren's syndrome, 15 percent of those with rheumatoid arthritis, and 22 percent of those with systemic lupus erythematosus have a secondary fibromyalgia.

LYME DISEASE

Since the mid-1970s, physicians have known that a deer-borne tick, *Ixodes dammini,* can infect people with a spirochete bacterium known as *Borrelia burgdorferi.* The disease was named for the area around Lyme, Connecticut, where it was first described; 90 percent of all cases are reported in the New England and mid-Atlantic regions.

Lyme disease is a complex malady. It presents in three stages. About one-third of tick bites are followed within a month by a distinct rash known as *erythema chronicum migrans.* Several weeks later, patients develop a generalized flu-like condition that may include joint swelling, muscle and joint aches, headache, sore throat, cough, fever, and swollen glands. If they are not treated with antibiotics (and infrequently if they have been treated), about 10 percent of the original group go on to a third stage in which potentially serious heart or nervous system involvement can develop.

What does fibromyalgia have to do with Lyme disease? First, a postinfectious fatigue/fibromyalgia syndrome ultimately afflicts a minority of Lyme disease patients. Second, many people who were told they had Lyme disease in fact had fibromyalgia. The reasoning is similar to what has been related about the Epstein-Barr virus. Some blood tests for Lyme disease are not very reliable for diagnosing the disease, and many patients who consult a doctor for fibromyalgia-like symptoms have evidence of prior exposure to the Lyme disease—including spirochete bacterium. Does this simply represent being in an endemic area where many residents have been exposed, or is the condition actually a postinfectious Lyme fibromyalgia? There is an important reason to try to determine this. Patients who have evidence of Lyme disease should receive a course of antibiotics in order to prevent the more serious third stage of the disease. However, this expensive and time-consuming therapy is rarely necessary. If a primary care physician is not sure what to do, rheumatology or infectious disease specialty evaluations may be useful.

REFLEX SYMPATHETIC DYSTROPHY

Reflex sympathetic dystrophy (RSD) can be induced by trauma, surgery, or certain drugs, or may occur spontaneously. A patient initially notices burning, tingling, and throbbing, sensitivity to touch or cold, and swelling of an arm or leg. A thorough examination usually demonstrates that both sides of the body are involved, although one side is more swollen than the other. The skin may be red or mottled. The affected extremity is painful to the touch and difficult to move. At first, a doctor may suspect a rheumatoid-like inflammatory arthritis. The swelling represents a form of neurogenic inflammation (see Chapter 3). In the second phase of RSD, the swelling becomes brawny and thicker, with pigment changes three to six months later. The numbness, burning, and tingling persist. After one or two years, muscle atrophy and wasting are evident in the affected limb, affected bones become osteoporotic (termed *Sudeck's atrophy*), and range of motion may be decreased. The swelling disappears, but a chronic pain syndrome with generalized fibromyalgia develops. A milder, regional RSD known as *shoulder-hand syndrome* is associated with a frozen or immobile shoulder.

RSD is a form of sympathetically mediated pain. Officially designated as a *complex regional pain syndrome*, it afflicts 1 person in 5,000.

Occurring when peripheral sensory receptors are oversensitized or outgoing sympathetic impulses are short-circuited to incoming sensory fibers, RSD can be a type of *causalgia,* consisting of sustained burning pain with allodynia, increased reaction to a stimulus, and dysfunction of autonomically mediated blood vessel tone. In RSD, chronic nociceptive stimulation produces sympathetic nervous system reactions (illustrated in Figure 11). This painful condition is very frustrating and difficult to treat. RSD probably represents 1–2 percent of fibromyalgia patients in a community rheumatology practice.

In its early phase, RSD should be managed aggressively with short courses of high-dose corticosteroids, vigorous mobilization, and physi-

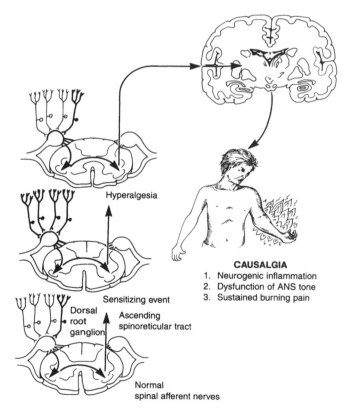

Hyperalgesia

CAUSALGIA
1. Neurogenic inflammation
2. Dysfunction of ANS tone
3. Sustained burning pain

Sensitizing event

Dorsal root ganglion

Ascending spinoreticular tract

Normal spinal afferent nerves

Fig. 11 *Reflex sympathetic dystrophy. Amplified musculoskeletal pain is complicated by ANS reactions that lead to severe burning, pain, and swelling.*

cal therapy. Once RSD has entered the second stage, some of its chronic features may be irreversible. In addition to fibromyalgia therapies, two additional aspects of RSD therapy need time and careful consideration. First, prolonged, aggressive physical therapy is helpful. Preferably, this should be prescribed in consultation with a physical medicine and re-habilitation specialist or orthopedist. Local steroid injections and sym-pathetic nervous system blockade are frequently helpful. Second, RSD patients may require narcotic pain medication in order to make it through the day, and a pain management consultation with follow-up may be advisable.

PREMENSTRUAL SYNDROME AND DYSMENORRHEA

The release of hormones, prostaglandins, and other chemicals along with serotonin dysfunction prior to the onset of menses can cause fluid retention, a sense of bloating, alterations in mood and behavior, and occasionally painful periods (dysmenorrhea). While most women ex-perience these cyclical alterations, 3–10 percent of American women have severe physical and psychological symptoms that interfere with their ability to function. They complain of irritability, tension, head-ache, backache, breast tenderness, depression, lack of energy, diffi-culty concentrating, a sleep disorder, and feeling "out of control." About 70 percent of women with fibromyalgia experience flares premenstru-ally, and the prevalence of fibromyalgia among those with more se-vere dysmenorrhea is increased. In addition to managing fibromyalgia, treating doctors frequently add an ibuprofen- or naproxen-containing anti-inflammatory agent to be taken a few days just before the onset of menstruation. Other women report relief when they take a mild di-uretic (water pill) for these few days as well.

CHRONIC PELVIC PAIN

As visceral structures, the urethra, bladder neck, vagina, and rectum are attached to striated, or voluntary muscles. Visceral receptors are usually fairly silent. When abnormally activated, they can cause chronic pelvic pain.

Irritable Bladder, or Female Urethral Syndrome

Among young women, urinary tract infections are extremely common. All too often, in order to make it convenient for the doctor and the patient, antibiotics are prescribed by telephone for symptoms and signs of burning with voiding, blood in the urine, or frequent urination. In an ideal world, antibiotics should be prescribed after a urine culture is obtained, and the prescription might be altered 48 to 72 hours later when the infecting organism has been grown and identified. Some patients have recurrent infections, and still others are on chronic antibiotic prophylactic therapy.

Within this population, a subgroup of young women fall through the cracks. They complain of intense pain with urination, and the urinalysis may show a few pus cells or red blood cells. The urine cultures are always negative, and mechanical problems such as a urethral stricture or neurogenic bladder are not present. Sometimes the pain seems to lessen with an antibiotic, although this is usually because doctors frequently add anesthetic medicines (e.g., phenazopyridine [Pyridium]) to the antibiotic, which diminishes discomfort while voiding. These patients have *female urethral syndrome,* which our group was the first to associate with fibromyalgia. Representing spasm of the muscles around the urethra, an irritable bladder is found in 10–15 percent of fibromyalgia patients. Its management consists of reassurance, avoiding antibiotics, phenazopyridine hydrochloride (Pyridium), and antispasmodics (e.g., oxybutynin, tolterodine [Ditropan, Detrol]). We have found that when muscle relaxants such as diazepam (Valium) or cyclobenzaprine (Flexeril) are taken for a few nights, urethral spasm usually abates for periods ranging from days to months.

Vulvodynia and Vaginismus

Seen in less than 5 percent of fibromyalgia patients, intense discomfort in the female genital tract can reflect a painful vulva (the visible external female genital area) without infection or other pathology (*vulvodynia*) or involuntary spasms of the vaginal muscles when entry is attempted (*vaginismus*). Many of these women have chronic, tense holding patterns that developed in childhood. Causes include abuse, traumatic toilet training, abnormal bowel habits, stress, dance training, pelvic trauma,

pelvic infectious inflammatory disease, pelvic trauma, and guilt surrounding sexual feelings. This results in painful intercourse and has
serious lifestyle implications. Many of these women also have female
urethral syndrome. Studies have shown that many women with vulvodynia or vaginismus have a history of sexual or physical abuse, a
rape experience, or psychological problems especially related to feelings of guilt, anger, fear, or loss of control. In addition to prescribing
medication to manage fibromyalgia, we advise our vulvodynia or
vaginismus patients to seek counseling with an understanding sex therapist and/or psychologist experienced in this sensitive area. Biofeedback to the pelvic floor musculature and/or botox injections into the
pelvic musculature ameliorates some of the symptoms.

Interstitial Cystitis

Interstitial cystitis could be considered a controversial condition because of its lack of a clear-cut definition. Classic interstitial cystitis is
defined as bladder and pelvic pain, frequency, and urinary urgency in
a patient with negative urine cultures. Associated with voiding hesi-
tancy, it worsens with menses and menopause. Cystoscopy reveals inflammation, blood, and frequently scarring when biopsy samples are

Table 9. *Fibromyalgia-associated conditions*

Condition	% who have fibromyalgia	% with fibromyalgia who have associated conditions
Chronic fatigue syndrome	50	50
Functional bowel	20	40
Autoimmune disease	10	2
Lyme disease	30	2
Reflex dystrophy	100	5
Premenstrual syndrome	10	50
Female urethral syndrome	10	12
Vulvodynia, vaginismus	50	5
Mitral valve prolapse	10	20
Tension headache	20	53
TMJ dysfunction	18	75
U.S. population	2	—

viewed under the microscope. The bladder muscle wall can be thick and vascular with superficial ulcerations, but the lining mucosa is friable and thin. Classic interstitial cystitis is seen in autoimmune diseases (especially lupus), after radiation therapy, and in patients who had chronic bladder infections in the past.

Unfortunately, some practitioners (particularly nonurologists) term what we call female urethral syndrome interstitial cystitis; others use the term loosely on the basis of the above-listed symptoms without cystoscopic confirmation. The bladder wall also has high levels of substance P. An increased percentage of patients who fall into the categories listed in this paragraph have fibromyalgia.

STEROID, HEROIN, ALCOHOL, OR COCAINE WITHDRAWAL

Corticosteroids are prescribed for a variety of inflammatory and allergic conditions ranging from asthma, ulcerative colitis, and sinus irritation to rheumatoid arthritis and lupus, and along with chemotherapy for certain malignancies. When steroids are taken for more than a few weeks, the skin becomes very sensitive to touch or pressure. It also becomes sensitive to small alterations in steroid doses. For example, if a patient is taking 15 mg of prednisone and the dose is reduced to 10 mg, the decrease in dose can produce a *steroid withdrawal fibromyalgia*. This is not classical fibromyalgia because if the dose stays at 10 mg, most of the fibromyalgia-like pain and spasm disappear within a few weeks. Long-term steroid administration is associated with secondary fibromyalgia by causing increased skin and soft tissue sensitivity.

Acute, transient circumstances in which a temporary fibromyalgia-like situation occurs are also found in patients withdrawing from alcohol, heroin, or cocaine.

TENSION HEADACHE SYNDROME, MITRAL VALVE PROLAPSE, AND OTHERS

Headaches are a common feature of fibromyalgia. Detailed histories indicate that many patients who seek neurologic consultation for tension headaches turn out to have fibromyalgia symptoms and signs. We discussed tension headaches and mitral valve prolapse in Chapter 4. Other syndromes associated with fibromyalgia include chronic hyperventilation, increased awareness of cardiac activity (palpitation sensations without mitral valve prolapse or cardiac abnormality), and globus hystericus (where patients continually complain of a lump in their throat).

CONTROVERSIAL SYNDROMES AND THEIR RELATIONSHIPS TO FIBROMYALGIA

Over the years, a variety of health professionals have developed terms or phrases to denote seemingly unique clinical combinations of symptoms and signs. A disorder or syndrome does not necessarily exist simply because it has been described in the medical literature. Some have stood the test of time, others overlap with syndromes described by different specialists, and additional terms may be favored by a single practitioner advocating a "cause." These conditions have overlapping features with fibromyalgia but are not yet regarded as full-blown, legitimate disorders by organized medicine.

Allergies and "Multiple Chemical Sensitivity" Syndrome

Self-reported environmental sensitivities are observed in 15 percent of Americans. From 3–7 percent of fibromyalgia patients report extreme sensitivity to enviromnental components, particularly cigarette smoke, noise, bright lights, cold temperatures, pollution, gas, paint, perfumes, solvent fumes, pesticides, auto exhaust, certain foods, and carpet smells. A study conducted by the National Institutes of Health documented that one-half to three-quarters of patients with chronic fatigue syndrome (CFS) complain of having many allergies and sensitivities.

Multiple chemical sensitivity syndrome is a controversial entity. Proponents of the syndrome explain that it is triggered by exposure to diverse chemicals at doses lower than those documented to cause adverse effects in humans. They further define the condition as being reproducible with repeated exposure of chemically unrelated multiple substances that can affect multiple organs and symptoms that improve when the incitants are removed. *Cacosmia* is the subjective sense of feeling ill from low levels of environmental chemical odors.

Cognitive impairment complaints are common. Interestingly, conventional allergy skin tests are usually normal.

About 5 percent of allergists call themselves *clinical ecologists* and attribute many of our nation's ills to environmental sensitivities. They use terms such as *chemically induced immune dysregulation, food allergies, leaky gut syndrome, allergic tension-fatigue syndrome, allergic toxemia, twentieth-century disease, ecologic illness,* or *yeast syndrome* to explain these conditions. This group is not recognized by organized medicine and has developed testing methodologies that are not endorsed by mainstream practitioners. The National Research Council and the American Medical Association have issued position papers stating that there is not enough evidence to recognize multiple chemical sensitivity as a clinical syndrome. Many highly respected allergy/immunology specialists believe that multiple chemical sensitivity syndrome is overdiagnosed; others do not think it exists. The American Academy of Allergy and Immunology, the American College of Physicians (to which most internists belong), and the American College of Occupational Medicine have issued position statements that the clinical ecology literature provides inadequate support for their beliefs and practices. In other words, double-blind, prospective trials (in which patients did not know what they were being tested for or treated with and half of whom received no treatment) have not borne out clinical ecology theories.

Most patients labeled as having multiple chemical sensitivity syndrome have nociceptive amplification as a form of fibromyalgia or CFS, while others have a primary psychological disturbance, primarily a panic/anxiety disorder, which may play a role in these complaints. Additionally, we have had patients whose symptoms and signs disappeared with antiallergy therapies. Some "mutiple chemical sensitivity" is not immunologic but is a form of hypervigilance that results from the ability of the olfactory neurons and the limbic system to amplify responses to chemicals in concert with a dysfunctioning ANS.

The most important issue in treating patients with environmental sensitivities and allergies is to make sure that they do not become so fearful of going outside and living normally that they become "environmental cripples."

A subset of patients with chemical sensitivity developed their condition, known as *sick building syndrome,* or *building-related illness,* after a defined exposure to microbes or allergens. Evaluating the structure's temperature, humidity, dust, formaldehyde, carbon monoxide, volatile, and organic compounds is usually revealing. Because their fibromyalgia-like conditions evolved in numerous individuals after exposure to specific chemicals found in structures, this group of patients usually has a better prognosis than the overall multiple chemical sensitivity group in general.

Patients diagnosed with multiple chemical sensitivity syndrome should have their fibromyalgia managed symptomatically. They should work closely with an allergist/immunologist once a primary psychiatric disorder has been ruled out or treatment has been initiated.

Gulf War Syndrome

A total of 697,000 U.S. soldiers served in the 1991 Persian Gulf War. A combination of symptoms characterized by fatigue (61 percent), joint pain (51 percent), nasal sinus congestion (51 percent), diarrhea (44 percent), joint stiffness, irritable colon, myalgias, cognitive impairment (all 41 percent), and headache (39 percent) was reported initially by 17,248 (2.5 percent) military personnel and some complaints ultimately by approximately 50,000 soldiers. When strict criteria were applied (symptoms starting two to three months after leaving the Persian Gulf with a duration of more than six months, other diseases having been ruled out), probably 3,000 military personnel had what has been called *Gulf War syndrome.* Gulf War syndrome may have been induced by giving combatants an insect repellent known as DEET in combination with pyridostigmine, an agent that minimizes the toxicity of nerve gas. Together, these drugs prolong acetylcholine activity and can produce some of the symptoms reported by the soldiers. Other mechanisms for Gulf War syndrome have also been proposed. Several well-documented reports found that 17–25 percent of Gulf War syndrome patients fulfilled the ACR criteria for fibromyalgia.

Siliconosis

This controversial condition is based on the premise that the silicone in breast implants can be broken down to silica or related products, which spread throughout the body. For over 50 years, silica has been known to stimulate the immune system. Among exposed gold and uranium miners, silica occasionally results in the formation of autoantibodies and a scleroderma- or lupus-like disorder 10–30 years after exposure. *Siliconosis,* a term coined by Dr. Gary Solomon at New York University in the early 1990s, could be its cousin seen in some patients with breast implants. Many siliconosis patients have a fibromyalgia-like condition with chronic fatigue, muscle and joint pain, swollen lymph glands, dry eyes, cognitive dysfunction, and difficulty swallowing, with or without the presence of autoantibodies. Other physicians have countered that silicone is not broken down to silica, and they believe that the role of these symptoms and illnesses is no different in women without implants. In the current litigious atmosphere, it will probably be several years before these claims are sorted out in a scientifically acceptable fashion.

Leaky Gut and "Yeast" Syndromes

Irritable bowel, spastic colitis, and functional bowel disease are recognized disorders of visceral hyperalgesia (increased pain sensitivity in internal structures), along with altered gut motility. Over the years, some homeopaths, naturopaths, and other alternative medicine practitioners have hypothesized that when too many substances pass through the lining of the small intestine, it becomes more permeable than usual. In other words, an overload of toxins or poisons is present that overwhelms the ability of the liver to detoxify them. As a consequence, inflammation and infections, as well as hormonal and neuromuscular changes, ensue.

Known as the *leaky gut syndrome,* this disorder has been held to cause *reactive hypoglycemia,* or low blood sugar, which in turn can induce palpitations, low blood pressure, and a feeling of faintness. Leaky gut syndrome has been claimed to be aggravated by aspirin- and ibuprofen-like products, food allergies, and yeast. Standard medical textbooks do not mention the existence of leaky gut syndrome, and most mainstream physicians believe that the majority of these patients have functional bowel or psychiatric disorders. However, our group has shown that fibromyalgia patients have increased intestinal bacterial overgrowth. The significance is not known at this time.

Candida hypersensitivity syndrome is a variant of the leaky gut syndrome, according to Dr. William Crook, a Tennessee family practitioner, who popularized the theories of Dr. C. Orian Truss in a 1983 bestseller, *The Yeast Connection: A Medical Breakthrough.* Yeast is a fungus known by the technical term *candida.* Verifiable yeast infections are present in healthy people, as well as being a complication of diabetes; pregnancy; progesterone, steroid, chemotherapy or antibiotic therapy; and altered immune states. Dr. Crook hypothesized that certain people develop hypersensitivity to a toxin released by yeast that exists naturally in the gastrointestinal tract, vagina, and respiratory tract. This, along with a lack of "good" bacteria, leads to a general feeling of ill health and to the same inflammatory, immune, hormonal, and neuromuscular changes attributed to leaky gut syndrome. Dr. Crook advocated a diet with carefully controlled sugar, wheat product, and yeast intake, attention to food allergies, nutritional supplements, and anti-yeast medication.

Unfortunately, no controlled trials in the peer review literature support his claim, and when anti-yeast medication was given in a double-blind fashion (where half of the patients unknowingly took a placebo), no differences were noted. Yeast antibody tests are available in many clinical laboratories but consistently fail to identify patients who are infected—only those who have been exposed, which is virtually all of us. The American Academy of Allergy and Immunology issued a position paper stating that "the concept (of a yeast connection) is speculative and unproven . . . elements of the proposed treatment program are potentially dangerous."

Arnold-Chiari (Chiari Malformation) Myelopathy

Some of our patients have asked us if they qualify for the "surgical cure" of fibromyalgia. Such a cure does not exist, but desperate individuals sometimes undergo an expensive, painful procedure promoted by a few advocates that in our experience does not help the syndrome. Syrinomyelia and Chiari malformations are congenital or acquired disorders of the upper spine involving compression of nerves. Parts of the cerebellum (back of the brain) herniate into the spinal column and compress the brainstem, which produces headaches, burning and shooting pains in the back and neck, fatigue, vertigo, hearing loss, blurred or double vision, and a staggering gait. As usually performed, CT or MR imaging of the neck and brain rarely show this condition unless special views are ordered. These seriously ill patients do not have fibromyalgia, but a compressive myelopathy that mimics it. They benefit from decompressive surgery, but the condition is relatively rare.

Some individuals with Chiari malformations have been *misdiagnosed* as having fibromyalgia. If your family doctor finds very brisk reflexes or a Babinski reflex on a routine examination and the above complaints are present, a Chiari workup is indicated. Nearly all patients with Chiari malformations have this easy to find neurologic testing abnormality. A recent study of fibromyalgia patients found no differences in abnormalities in brain and spine imaging consistent with Chiari malformations compared with a control group. Many healthy people (and patients with fibromyalgia) have slight imaging abnormalities suggesting an asymptomatic, mild Chiari-like compression.

Mercury Amalgams

The use of mercury-silver amalgam fillings in the mouth has been held to produce chronic fatigue, headaches, cognitive dysfunction, and muscle and joint aches. Although the American Dental Association considers mercury amalgams to be a safe, effective method of tooth restoration, there may be an extremely small group of patients who are sensitive to this product. When patients with fibromyalgia raise this question, I reply that in 20 years of practice only one patient of mine (out of 12,000 seen) has had all symptoms disappear with the removal of mercury amalgam fillings.

Controversial Syndromes: Summing Up

If you have been diagnosed as having multiple chemical sensitivity syndrome, Gulf War syndrome, siliconosis, a leaky gut with or without yeast infection, mercury amalgam toxicity, or interstitial cystitis, be aware that these diagnoses are controversial and may not truly exist. Before initiating expensive, time-consuming, toxic, or lifestyle-altering therapies that are unproven, make sure that your treating physicians agree on the best course of action to take. Or at least, look before you leap!

7
The Fibromyalgia Consultation and Differential Diagnosis

Fibromyalgia is usually a diagnosis of exclusion. Often poorly understood by some primary care physicians, its diagnosis is often delayed. Even though in one survey up to 10 percent of general medical visits involve a complaint of generalized musculoskeletal pain, the diagnosis was made only after patients saw a mean of 3.5 doctors. This chapter will take you through the workup that establishes the definitive diagnosis and eliminates other possible explanations for the patient's complaints.

WHO SHOULD BE THE FIBROMYALGIA CONSULTANT AND HOW CAN THE PATIENT PREPARE FOR THE VISIT?

Suppose that you are suspected of having fibromyalgia, and a primary care physician has referred you to a fibromyalgia consultant (usually a rheumatologist but sometimes an internist, physiatrist, neurologist, orthopedist, or osteopath) to confirm the diagnosis and make management suggestions. Is any sort of advanced preparation advisable? Yes. Bring copies of outside records and previous test results or workups to the consultant. If you have more than a few complaints or are taking more than a few medications, a summary list is useful. The evaluation will consist of an interview, or history, physical examination, diagnostic laboratory tests, and possibly imaging studies (X-rays, scans, etc.). Once all the observations and test results are in, the doctor will discuss the findings with you—perhaps at the time of the visit, by telephone after the initial meeting, or in a follow-up visit.

MUST BLOOD BE DRAWN OR URINE EXAMINED?

A history and physical examination may suggest the diagnosis of fibromyalgia, but in order to make sure that other disorders with complaints and physical findings similar to those of fibromyalgia are not present, it is necessary to perform blood laboratory tests.

When a patient arrives at an internist's or family practitioner's office for a general medical evaluation, it usually includes what doctors refer to as *screening laboratory tests*. In other words, by obtaining a blood count, urine test, and blood chemistry panel, abnormalities can be detected in 90 percent of individuals with serious medical problems.

WHAT ABOUT IMAGING STUDIES OR ELECTRICAL EVALUATIONS?

When evaluating a potential fibromyalgia patient, I usually obtain a chest X-ray and electrocardiogram (EKG) of the heart if one has not been done recently. These are also inexpensive and safe procedures that rule out potentially important causes of chest area pains, palpitations, and shortness of breath.

In certain circumstances, additional blood testing may be useful. Autoimmune blood tests consisting of an ANA or rheumatoid factor screen for systemic lupus and rheumatoid arthritis may be necessary. If these tests are positive, as they are in a small number of fibromyalgia patients, specific additional ANA panels can be obtained to confirm the diagnosis. Fibromyalgia patients frequently complain of numbness, tingling, and burning. The doctor may want to get X-rays (and, if abnormal, an MRI or computed tomography [CT] scan) of the neck or low back to make sure that a bone spur or herniated disc is not causing these symptoms. An electromyogram (EMG) can also diagnose herniated discs or indicate if numbness is from carpal tunnel syndrome, diabetes, or an inflammatory process. In difficult cases, a spinal X-ray performed after injecting dye into the spinal column, known as a *myelogram,* usually determines if a herniated disc is present. Bone scans can look for tumors or inflammation. Sleep EEGs (polysomnography) may be ordered if it is important to document a physiologic basis for complaints of unrefreshing sleep.

There are additional blood tests, imaging, and electrical studies that are inexpensive and useful and may be appropriate in specific situations.

ARE YOU SURE IT'S REALLY FIBROMYALGIA?

Fibromyalgia can seem to be working in concert with other diseases. For example, untreated inflammation associated with an autoimmune disease (such as rheumatoid arthritis or systemic lupus erythematosus), other forms of inflammatory arthritis (such as ankylosing spondylitis), or a chest disease known as *sarcoidosis* are associated with coexisting fibromyalgia. Withdrawal from or tapering of medications such as corticosteroids typically precipitates or aggravates fibromyalgia.

Many disorders interact with or can be mistaken for fibromyalgia. They are reviewed here, as well as in other parts of this book, and listed in Table 10.

Table 10. *Common conditions and disorders that can mimic fibromyalgia*

Hormonal imbalances
    Menstrual disorders
    Low thyroid, high parathyroid levels
    Pregnancy
    Adrenal insufficiency
    Diabetes
    Menopause
Infections
    Bacteria
    Viruses
    Fungi
    Parasites
Musculoskeletal or autoimmune disorders
    Rheumatoid arthritis
    Ankylosing spondylitis in females
    Seronegative spondyloarthropathies
    Lyme disease
    Systemic lupus erythematosus
    Palindromic rheumatism
    Inflammatory bowel disease
    Polymyalgia rheumatica
Neurologic disease
    Multiple sclerosis
    Myasthenia gravis
Malignancy
Substance abuse
Malnutrition
Primary psychiatric disorders
Allergies

Hormonal Imbalances

Low *thyroid* levels, or *hypothyroidism* can be mistaken for fibromyalgia. Blood T_3, T_4, and TSH tests readily and inexpensively differentiate these disorders. *Parathyroid tumors* or adenomas raise blood calcium levels and cause aching, weakness, and palpitations. The parathyroid gland overlies the thyroid, and disorders of this gland are detected by measuring calcium, phosphorus, and Parathormone blood levels. *Adrenal glands* overlie the kidney and make cortisone. Adrenal insufficiency (Addison's disease) or adrenal overactivity (Cushing's disease) can modulate fibromyalgia symptoms. *Diabetics* with peripheral nerve disease complain of numbness and tingling. If their sugar levels are too high or too low, they complain of fatigue, palpitations, and weakness.

Hormonal disorders produce fatigue, aching, and weakness. *Premenstrual syndrome (PMS)* frequently aggravates fibromyalgia symptoms. *Menopause* can improve fibromyalgia, but early menopausal symptoms can mimic and aggravate the syndrome. Irregular periods, use of birth control pills, and painful periods may produce symptoms of bloating, fatigue, and aching. It is also important to make sure that new fibromyalgia-like symptoms are not in fact an early *pregnancy*.

Infections

Bacteria, viruses, fungi, parasites, and other microbes infect the body and produce a variety of systemic reactions, including fatigue, malaise, fevers, swollen glands, rashes, joint pain, shortness of breath, abdominal pain, and difficulty thinking clearly. Infections and fibromyalgia can interact in three different ways: postinfectious fatigue syndromes can cause fibromyalgia and chronic fatigue syndrome, fibromyalgia may be mistaken for infection and vice versa, and infections can aggravate fibromyalgia.

A doctor can screen for infections with the workup reviewed in the previous chapter but may need additional tests. These may include cultures of blood, urine, sputum, stool, bone marrow, skin lesions, spinal fluid, pleural fluid, or whatever bodily tissues are accessible, and serum antibody levels to organisms to ascertain prior or current exposure. Sometimes, doctors perform skin tests (such as a tuberculosis skin test) or order scans to identify infected areas. Infections should be promptly identified and treated.

Musculoskeletal Disorders

As mentioned earlier, 7–22 percent of patients with autoimmune diseases have secondary fibromyalgia and may be mistakenly diagnosed as having the syndrome. Early *rheumatoid arthritis* sometimes appears fibromyalgia-like before it settles in the hands and feet and causes joint swelling. *Systemic lupus erythematosus* is commonly misdiagnosed as fibromyalgia because overlapping fatigue, aching, and cognitive impairment symptoms can be confusing. Ten million Americans have a positive ANA, which is almost always seen in lupus, but only one million Americans have lupus. Therefore, patients who present to a rheumatologist with a positive ANA and nonspecific symptoms often go through a workup to rule out lupus, which may include obtaining muscle enzymes, inflammatory indices such as sedimentation rate, skin biopsy specimens, bone scans, and detailed autoantibody blood testing. *Polymyositis* is an inflammatory muscle disease differentiated from fibromyalgia by elevation of the muscle enzyme creatine phosphokinase in blood testing.

Rheumatoid variants such as *ankylosing spondylitis, psoriatic arthritis, arthritis of inflammatory bowel disease,* and *reactive arthritis* may be hard to distinguish from fibromyalgia since they are often only intermittently inflammatory. Many rheumatoid variant patients have a positive blood test for a marker known as HLA-B27. *Palindromic rheumatism* presents as a prerheumatoid arthritis, prelupus-like condition, with infrequent physical findings of joint swelling and symptoms of aching and fatigue. *Polymyalgia rheumatica* is seen in older patients who have aching in their shoulder and hip areas; it is usually easy to differentiate from fibromyalgia since the blood sedimentation rate is elevated.

Hypermobility syndromes and *work overuse syndromes* may be misdiagnosed as fibromyalgia but are associated with regional myofascial syndromes, as are *osteoarthritis, spinal stenosis,* and *disc problems* in the cervical and lumbar spines. Most people in their 40s and 50s have nonspecific abnormalities on X-rays or CT or MRI scans, and sometimes low back pain or neck pain is interpreted as a herniated disc when it is really due to fibromyalgia. Low back pain costs Americans $24 billion a year. Eighty percent of this amount is incurred by 5 percent of those with low back pain, in some of whom the diagnosis of fibromyalgia is overlooked.

Neurologic Disease

Patients with early forms of *multiple sclerosis* and *myasthenia gravis* complain of numbness, aching, fatigue, weakness, and difficulty thinking clearly without dramatic physical findings. Unlike fibromyalgia, multiple sclerosis is characterized by MRI and spinal fluid abnormalities, and myasthenia gravis is marked by abnormal electrical studies and positive antibody tests. To further confuse the issue, secondary fibromyalgia accompanies neurologic disease in up to 20 percent of these patients. Primary muscle or nerve disorders associated with complaints of numbness, tingling, or burning can be differentiated from fibromyalgia by EMG and nerve conduction studies, as well as by various forms of spinal imaging. Nerve or muscle biopsies are occasionally recommended to clarify the diagnosis.

Malignancies

Patients with cancer make a variety of extra chemicals, many of which cause systemic symptoms, including fatigue, aching, and weakness, that resemble fibromyalgia complaints. These *paraneoplastic* features of a tumor usually disappear with treatment including chemotherapy, radiation therapy, and surgery. Steroids frequently are used along with chemotherapy, and disease onset and/or changes can produce fibromyalgia. Selected drugs used to treat cancer, such as *alpha-interferon* (for leukemia) or *interleukin-2* (e.g., for melanoma or kidney cancer) may induce fibromyalgia-like symptoms that last for weeks to months. Healthy-appearing young women with early stages of *Hodgkin's disease* and other *lymphomas* initially have been diagnosed incorrectly as having fibromyalgia.

Substance Abuse and Malnutrition

Our society provides many means—legal and otherwise—to obtain agents that can produce or alleviate fatigue. Caffeine is an addictive chemical in coffee, tea, headache formulas (e.g., Excedrin, Fiorinal), and cola beverages that can increase the heart rate. People who are dependent on caffeine develop fatigue and palpitations or withdrawal symptoms when they are deprived of it for a day or two. Many of these individuals take diet pills or "uppers" to manage fatigue, which can also lead to appetite loss, weight loss, and malnutrition. The number of patients who complain of profound fatigue and do not realize (or deny) that it could be due to taking high doses of prescription painkillers such as Vicodin, codeine, Darvon, or Percocet is amazing. Alcohol, cocaine, and heroin abuse are common causes of fatigue, but dependence on pain medicine is very common. Sudden withdrawal of any of these substances is associated with pain amplification.

FIBROMYALGIA SUBSETS: CHILDHOOD AND ADOLESCENCE

Whereas fibromyalgia is present in 2 percent of adults and is the third or fourth most common reason for seeking a rheumatology consultation, it is the twelfth most common reason for seeking a pediatric rheumatology evaluation. Pediatric rheumatologists see a new child or adolescent with fibromyalgia just a few times a year. There are probably fewer than 10,000 children in the United States with the syndrome, 90 percent of whom are adolescents. This has led some investigators to speculate that a hormonal connection may be very important. In addition to its relative rarity, preadult fibromyalgia is different from adult fibromyalgia. How so? It differs in two ways: reflex sympathetic dystrophy (RSD) and a typical psychiatric profile.

Few centers have much experience with childhood fibromyalgia, but studies from Children's Hospital of Los Angeles suggest that a subset of adolescents with fibromyalgia fit a specific profile. An example could be a 10- to 15-year-old girl who has grown up as a "perfect, model" child, never complains, and has perfectionistic tendencies and excellent grades in school. They appear mature beyond their years, and meet the needs of others at their own expense. Mom frequently acts as the spokesperson at the rheumatology consultation.

A seemingly trivial sports injury or emotional event (e.g., a move, divorce, change in nuclear family, change in school or friends) can be followed by widespread pain and fatigue. Splinting or casting the injured area is of no benefit and "growing pains" simply don't get better. Additionally, reflex sympathetic dystrophy with swelling of both upper extremities (more severe on one side than on the other), inability to move an arm or shoulder, and mottling changes in the skin is often present. RSD is found in 1–10 percent of adult fibromyalgia patients but is seen in up to 20 percent of adolescents. Adolescents with severe growing pains, disturbed sleep, irritable colon, attention deficit, and hypermobile (very limber) joints frequently develop full-blown fibromyalgia in adulthood.

Unlike adult fibromyalgia, the juvenile syndrome responds only minimally to tricyclic antidepressants and pain medication. The best results correlate with intensive, vigorous physical therapy and exercise, steroid injections to affected areas or intermittent courses of oral steroids, and psychological support. Even though the presentation of fibromyalgia in young people is more severe than in adults, children and adolescents have a better prognosis than many adults. If the treatment program outlined above is aggressively pursued, 80 percent of young patients have substantial resolution of the syndrome within two to three years.

FIBROMYALGIA IN THE ELDERLY

As patients with long-standing fibromyalgia age, the syndrome usually persists. Many female patients report that menopause modestly decreases their symptoms. But can people over the age of 65 develop fibromyalgia-like symptoms? Since this is an unusual event, the differential diagnosis reviewed earlier in this chapter should be considered. This applies especially to hypothyroidism, Sjogren's syndrome (dry eyes, dry mouth, aching, and fatigue), rheumatoid arthritis, occult malignancy, and polymyalgia rheumatica. A normal sedimentation rate, negative ANA, negative rheumatoid factor, and normal TSH (thyroid test) usually allow doctors to make a definitive diagnosis of fibromyalgia. Studies of patients with older-onset fibromyalgia show fewer functional symptoms such as anxiety, stress, or unrefreshed sleep and more musculoskeletal complaints than their younger counterparts. Polymyalgia rheumatica is far more common than late-onset fibromyalgia. It presents with aching in the upper back, neck, buttocks, or thighs, along with a markedly elevated sedimentation rate. Many healthy older people have modestly elevated sedimentation rates. As a consequence, up to 40 percent of late-onset fibromyalgia patients in one survey were given corticosteroids before a correct diagnosis was made. Older-onset fibromyalgia is managed the same way as in younger adults. Finally, joint and muscle aches can be symptomatic of primary depression; this possibility always warrants careful consideration.

SUMMING UP

Fibromyalgia is a diagnosis of exclusion. Serious and treatable disorders with overlapping symptoms and signs should be ruled out before patients are convinced and the doctor feels comfortable with the diagnosis. If a patient has fibromyalgia secondary to one of several disorders, it won't get better until the primary or underlying disease is addressed. Doctors try their best, but the patient's symptoms, signs, and physical findings can be subtle and don't always lead directly to a diagnosis of fibromyalgia.

8

I'm Not Crazy!

"You look fine, and I can't find anything wrong with you. Maybe you're just depressed or stressed out." Nearly all of my patients have heard this before. And they start to wonder: Am I really crazy? How could it all be in my mind? This chapter will summarize the behavioral surveys that rheumatologists and psychiatrists have performed on fibromyalgia patients.

DO I HURT BECAUSE I'M DEPRESSED OR AM I DEPRESSED BECAUSE I HURT?

Is fibromyalgia a manifestation of depression or the reverse? Well-designed studies have addressed this issue, but many used different methods, populations, ethnic groupings, referral sources, and geographical distributions. In any case, the results were reasonably similar. On average, these studies showed that about 18 percent of fibromyalgia patients have evidence of a major depression at any office visit and 58 percent have a history of major depression in their lifetime. What does this mean? *At any point in time, the overwhelming majority of fibromyalgia patients are not seriously depressed.* And if they are depressed, it's usually because they do not feel well. This condition is called *reactive depression* and is reversible with treatment, as opposed to *endogenous depression,* which is caused by chemical imbalances and is much harder to treat. A well-designed study of depressed patients demonstrated that fewer than 10 percent had two or more tender points.

WHICH FACTORS ARE MORE COMMON IN FIBROMYALGIA PATIENTS THAN IN THOSE WITHOUT THE DISORDER?

Studies conducted in the last few years show that fibromyalgia patients have a significantly increased risk of having a history of sexual, physical, or drug abuse, eating disorders, mood disorders, attention deficit disorder, phobias (unrealistic fears), panic, anxiety, somatization, and a family history of depression or alcoholism. They also show that fibromyalgia patients cope less well with daily problems than others and are more susceptible to psychological stress. We have already shown that psychological stress can lower the pain threshold. Certain studies also suggest that there is more *alexithymia,* a longstanding personality disorder with generalized and localized complaints in individuals who cannot express their underlying psychological conflicts. As a consequence, some behavioral experts have proposed that fibromyalgia is an *affective spectrum disorder* in which a primary psychiatric disorder with a possibly inherited abnormality leads to pain amplification and fibromyalgia-related complaints.

These studies promoted an intense debate among fibromyalgia experts as to whether fibromyalgia is a manifestation of a *psychological* disturbance or a *physiological* disorder of pain amplification. We strongly believe that the latter explanation is more accurate. Why do we feel so strongly? First, biochemical abnormalities (e.g., increased substance P level in spinal fluid) have been found in fibromyalgia that do not correlate with behavioral abnormalities. Second, fibromyalgia frequently occurs in conditions such as scoliosis, which have never been associated with any behavioral disorders. Third, all of the behavioral surveys supporting an affective spectrum disorder were performed at university medical centers and do not reflect what an internist or family physician sees in a community fibromyalgia population practice. For example, sexual abuse may be one of *many* triggers or aggravating factors of fibromyalgia syndrome, but it is seen in a small number of patients with the syndrome. For most patients followed in a community practice, the syndrome is not serious enough for them to be referred to a specialist. Specialists generally deal with more severe cases, which skews their study results. A landmark study by Dr. Larry Bradley at the University of Alabama has clearly proven this point. *Though more patients with fibromyalgia have a history of psychosocial distress than patients with some other musculoskeletal conditions, this does not explain why a majority of individuals with fibromyalgia have no significant psychosocial distress.* If an affective spectrum and a somatization model do not accurately fit fibromyalgia, what does? Dr. Muhammed Yunus has recognized that there are many overlapping features among fibromyalgia, migraine, irritable colon, and tension headaches, for example. He has proposed that fibromyalgia is a *central sensitization syndrome (CSS)*, with an emphasis on chronic neuromuscular pain. Excluding all psychiatric diagnoses, Dr. Yunus and many of his colleagues now feel that fibromyalgia should be studied using the biomedical model. While agreeing that CSS is influenced by factors that govern psychological behavior, such as personality, mood, and attitude, the CSS model stresses that neurotransmitters are capable of biologically altering pain perception. Figure 12 demonstrates some of these interactions.

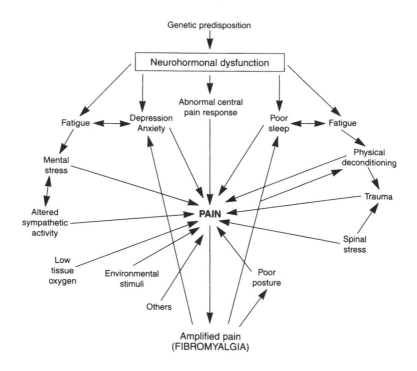

Fig. 12 *How chemicals associated with behavior biologically influence pain.*

FIBROMYALGIA PERSONALITY PROFILES

In the morning she was asked how she slept. "Oh terribly badly!" said the Princess. "I have scarcely shut my eyes the whole night. Heaven only knows what was in the bed, but I was lying on something hard, so that I am black and blue all over." Nobody but a real princess could be as sensitive as that. So the prince took her for his wife, for now he knew he had a real princess.

Hans Christian Andersen (1805–1875)
The Princess and the Pea, 1835

In our opinion, patients with fibromyalgia tend to have several personality profiles. At least half with the syndrome are females, aged 20–60, who have above average intelligence. They display perfectionistic tendencies, are efficient, well groomed, like to be organized, in control, and often make lists. An inciting event such as infection, trauma, new work responsibilities, or family pressures or stresses upset a delicate balance. Because they fear failure, rejection, or feel guilty due to the increasing difficultly in maintaining their current life styles and activities, a preexisting mild, chronic anxiety gets worse. This makes it difficult to sleep and ultimately leads to neuromuscular pain. Because it's harder to be as industrious, responsible, reliable, functional, and trustworthy as before and they seek favorable recognition, their anxiety worsens and pain increases. Several studies have shown that mild anxiety was present in 50–75 percent before the syndrome was diagnosed.

Other personality profiles may be present. Up to 20 percent of university-based fibromyalgia patients may have posttraumatic stress disorder (PTSD, see below), 20 percent severe emotional neglect and/or abuse, 20 percent chronic depression, and 5 percent panic disorders.

Posttraumatic Stress Disorder (PTSD)

Increased pain levels, emotional distress, varying degrees of disability, and interference with function are present in up to 20 percent of severe fibromyalgia patients at tertiary centers. Usually brought on by a specific traumatic event (e.g., death of a loved one), or continuous unpleasant circumstances (e.g., a tour of duty during the Afghan War), PTSD is associated with nightmares, recurrent and intensive recollections, and avoidance of thoughts and activities associated with the traumatic event or events. PTSD patients are easily aroused and display hypervigilance relating to fear and pain catastrophizing. They tend to be more aware of normal bodily sensations such as perception or sensitivity to noises, light, and heartbeats and frequently complain of dizziness.

CONDITIONS FIBROMYALGIA PATIENTS DO NOT HAVE THAT REQUIRE DIFFERENTIATION

There are other conditions that some doctors confuse with fibromyalgia, and several surveys cited above show that patients generally do *not* have them.

Hypochondriacs have an excessive fear of having a serious disease based on misinterpretation of one or more bodily symptoms and signs. They believe normal bodily sensations such as heartbeats and peristalsis represent a medical disorder. Nearly all fibromyalgia patients want to get well and accept reassurance that they are not seriously ill.

The psychiatric definition of *hysteria* differs from the common perception that these are individuals who are prone to ranting or raving. Hysterical patients complain of neurologic or body deficits that are not real and display a lack of concern (*la belle indifference*) or act blase about them. These conversion reactions involve statements that they cannot see, hear, or talk, or are paralyzed. An example would be a soldier in battle who reports that he cannot move his legs.

Patients who claim that they "hurt all over" but lack fibromyalgia tender points and have changing stories with inappropriate or inconsistent responses have a fictitious disease known as *psychogenic rheumatism.* These patients have serious emotional problems, and their complaints satisfy the psychological need for attention. Some are psychotic, or have lost touch with reality. Their stories make no biologic sense. The classic example is the patient who complains that "I hurt on the left side of my body, from the top of my head to the bottom of my toe." Anatomically, this is impossible since the nerve supply of these areas crosses the spinal cord at the neck and the head would hurt on the opposite side. Tender points are not found on examination, and no arthritis or muscle-focused therapies ever work. *Malingering,* or producing symptoms and signs for external gain, is not a feature of fibromyalgia.

Sometimes we encounter patients who are engrossed with themselves. They express excessive concern or fear of having a defect in appearance, a condition termed *body dysmorphic disorder*. These patients obsess over every blemish or bruise. Studies have shown no correlation between this behavior pattern and fibromyalgia.

Many doctors think that most fibromyalgia patients have perfectionistic tendencies. After all, many new fibromyalgia patients came to us with a neatly typed, detailed medical history and list of complaints. *Obsessive-compulsive personality disorder,* consists of a preoccupation with orderliness, perfectionism, and mental and interpersonal control at the expense of flexibility, openness, and efficiency. The bottom line is that perfectionism as part of obsessive-compulsive personality disorder is not more common, but perfectionistic tendencies may be.

SUMMING UP

Patients with fibromyalgia are not crazy and are infrequently depressed. They tend to experience more psychological distress, mild chronic anxiety, and psychosocial disruption. These manifestations are often associated with perfectioninstic tendencies and hypervigilance of normal bodily sensations. A biomedical model, wherein a biologic or physiologic response to pain influences psychologic well-being is the appropriate way to view fibromyalgia.

9

How to Help Yourself without Taking Medicine

Although there is no cure for fibromyalgia, patients can initiate numerous changes and make adjustments that improve their sense of well-being. Simply stated, there are things patients can do without spending money or seeing a healthcare provider. Demonstrating a certain amount of control over the syndrome also improves self-esteem and instills a sense of self-worth.

VITAMINS AND FOOD FOR THOUGHT: IS THERE A FIBROMYALGIA DIET?

Even though certain general dietary principles allow fibromyalgia patients to feel better, there is no "fibromyalgia diet." No specific food regimens or supplements have ever been shown in any published, controlled study to be helpful for fibromyalgia despite the observation that "arthritis diet" books are a multimillion-dollar-a-year industry.

How can we explain this discrepancy? First, people feel better when they eat healthy foods. Most arthritis diet books urge patients to eat three well-balanced meals a day and caution against overeating. Many recommend having the main meal at midday; heavy, late-evening dinners don't give the body enough time to burn off calories and are associated with bedtime esophageal spasm or heartburn. Similarly, consuming alcohol, nicotine, or caffeine (in the form of coffee, tea, or even chocolate) at a late dinner can make it harder to get a good night's sleep. Alcohol, in particular, should not be used as a painkiller. In turn, poor sleep can increase musculoskeletal pain. An acceptable healthy balance of proteins, carbohydrates, and fats can also increase energy and fight fatigue.

What about vitamins? As people always on the go, Americans tend to settle for the convenience of quick-to-prepare, easy-to-consume refined, processed foods that are relatively deficient in vitamins and minerals. Multivitamin and mineral supplements can be useful additions for those who don't have time or are unable to prepare well-balanced meals. Most vitamins, herbs, minerals, and supplements added to multivitamins are harmless, but some are occasionally associated with allergic reactions.

Food sensitivity plays a role in less than 10 percent of our fibromyalgia patients. Within this group, different foods affect people differently. For example, some fibromyalgia patients feel better when they eat fish, while others hurt more. Some practitioners believe that carbohydrates increase serotonin levels, essential fatty acids diminish fatigue, and proteins improve mental alertness. Others place patients on a hypoglycemic/yeast elimination diet consisting of small, frequent meals, along with carbohydrate and wheat product restrictions. We neither endorse nor refute any diet or food regimen for fibromyalgia, since none have been studied in a scientifically acceptable fashion. Thus, we have no admonitions for fibromyalgia patients regarding specific food groups.

ARE THERE MORE REASONS WHY SMOKING IS BAD?

Don't smoke. It's not only bad for obvious reasons, but it also aggravates fibromyalgia. Nicotine is a stimulant, which can make it harder to sleep at night. Cigarettes induce hyperreactivity in airways in the lung, cause wheezing, and decrease stamina. Over time, smoking accelerates atherosclerosis, or hardening of the arteries, which diminishes the amount of oxygen delivered to muscles; this, in turn, can cause pain. Dr. Yunus at the University of Illinois has demonstrated that smokers with fibromyalgia have lower pain thresholds and more sleep problems than nonsmokers. Nicotine withdrawal has been associated with muscle spasms. Finally, vascular constriction or spasm caused by abnormal functioning of the ANS, observed in 30–40 percent of fibromyalgia patients, is worsened by smoking and leads to increased numbness, burning, and tingling.

In other words, there are absolutely no healthy reasons to smoke!

CAN FIBROMYALGIA BE BLAMED
ON THE WEATHER?

There is no question about it, nearly all patients feel that climate influences their fibromyalgia. In one survey, 66 percent of fibromyalgia patients related that they were affected by weather changes: 78 percent preferred warm weather, 79 percent believed that cold weather made them feel worse, and 60 percent did not like humidity. A variety of studies have suggested that musculoskeletal stiffness, achiness, and pain are aggravated by *changes* in barometric pressure. Fibromyalgia symptoms can be aggravated when the weather shifts from hot to cold or from wet to dry. A consistent climate is associated with fewer musculoskeletal symptoms. For instance, Hawaii theoretically has the perfect climate for fibromyalgia patients since it is usually within 4 degrees of 83° F and humid year round. However, before contacting a realtor, it's important to realize that this does not allow for changes in barometric pressure from walking into and out of air-conditioned buildings all day. What's the best way to deal with changes in climate? Don't panic or get upset if it takes a few days to acclimatize when traveling or if the weather changes.

Fibromyalgia patients living in northern climates are especially susceptible to a condition known as *seasonal affective disorder.* Light deprivation during the winter predisposes one to depression and fatigue. This can lead to decreased energy, productivity, motivation, libido, patience, and the ability to focus one's thoughts. Bright lights or a midwinter trip to southern California, Arizona, or Florida can help break this form of emotional paralysis.

BUT I'M SO TIRED!

Fatigue is a significant complaint in 75–80 percent of fibromyalgia patients. It can destroy relationships, lower self-esteem, and cause other people to accuse one of "making it up" since fibromyalgia patients generally look healthy. There are many things that can be done before considering medication. Once other medical problems that cause fatigue are ruled out, there are better ways to manage daily activities.

First, is the patient taking prescription medications (especially muscle relaxants) during the day that make them tired? Can alcohol or illicit drug use be a factor? The fibromyalgia patient should avoid daytime napping, after the early afternoon; otherwise it's harder to sleep at night. Many patients have overextended lives and, before becoming ill, were intensely active and overinvolved. Perfectionistic (but not obsessive) tendencies also can lead to fatigue since these individuals push to accomplish more than they are really able to do. It's important to establish realistic goals.

Here are a few tips on how to overcome fatigue. Most important, learn the concept of pacing. Be busy for a couple of hours in the morning and then take a 15- to 20-minute break. Engage in activities for another two hours and eat a leisurely lunch. Alternating periods of activity with rest times allow most fibromyalgia patients to be as productive as healthy people. Don't stay in bed all day trying to conserve energy. This can lead to depression, premature osteoporosis, atrophy of the muscles, flexion contractures, and *increased* pain over time because poor conditioning prevents muscles from getting enough oxygen.

If fatigue is an overwhelming problem, adopt a strategy to deal with it. First, get a good night's sleep and embark on a conditioning program. Plan ahead and try to accomplish only what is really important. Learn to have certain responsibilities handled by others and limit commitments. Within the confines of the pacing concept, learn to manage time, use energy wisely, and perform tasks requiring the greatest amount of focusing and energy at the time of day when functioning best. Many fibromyalgia patients have a midday "window" of feeling better—for example, from 10:00 A.M. to 2:00 P.M. Remember, there are many things that alleviate fatigue short of taking medicine.

I DON'T SLEEP WELL!

A good night's sleep is critical to overcoming fibromyalgia. Sleep heals our muscles and decreases daytime fatigue. Over 75 percent of fibromyalgia patients report significant sleep problems.

Before considering a prescription sleep aid, there are many things that can be done to improve the sleep environment. First, take a look at the bedroom. Is the bed comfortable, the mattress firm, and the pillows suitable? A cervical pillow (our favorite is the Wal-Pil-O) reduces neck strain because it is shaped to support the neck. The room should be quiet and comfortable in temperature with a climate control system that keeps it neither too hot nor too cold. Don't let pets into the bedroom. Don't sleep with children. Don't exercise vigorously after dinner. And allow the room to become dark before going to bed.

Start preparing for a good night's sleep early in the day. Have a regular bedtime and wake up time. Don't nap after early afternoon. Don't drink a lot of fluids or take diuretics in the evening. Avoid caffeine, tobacco, alcohol, or a spicy or large meal too close to bedtime. On the other hand, don't starve, since hunger can also interfere with sleep. Use the hour before lights out to prepare for sleep. Think pleasing thoughts and practice slow, deep breathing. Soft music or relaxation tapes promote a restful mindset. Soak in a hot tub or take a hot shower and mentally close the day. Try not to read or listen to anything disturbing.

When the lights are turned out, one should fall asleep in 15–20 minutes. Falling asleep in less than five minutes suggests a state of sleep deprivation; on the other hand, if 30 minutes have elapsed, get up, since it's not time to sleep. With fibromyalgia, pain can make it difficult to fall or stay asleep, and patients need all the help they can muster. It may be more comfortable to lie on the back or side, or place a pillow under the knees to ease pressure on the lower back. If it's cold, consider using an electric blanket. Once asleep, try to sleep enough to feel refreshed in the morning. Make sure bed partners do not snore to the point of interfering with needed rest. Don't keep the television or radio on. If you awaken at 3:00 A.M. and cannot sleep, get up and putter. The problem should take care of itself within a few nights.

These routines are inexpensive and easy to carry out. Many fibromyalgia patients can overcome sleep problems without medication if they focus attention on their sleep environments.

DOCTOR, I'M IN PAIN!

Pain is a natural sensation that is an unavoidable feature of fibromyalgia. Don't let it be controlling—learn to control it. In pain amplification syndromes such as fibromyalgia, distractions make us less aware of discomfort. Whether we are listening to music, driving a car, watching a movie, or performing work activities, pain perception is lessened when we don't concentrate on it. Biofeedback, meditation, and other techniques help send healing messages to painful areas. Fibromyalgia pain is never caused by and does not lead to crippling deformities. It's impossible to hurt yourself while "walking through the pain" by sublimating the sensation.

MAKING A HOUSE A HOME

Fibromyalgia may try to control the patient, but one way of fighting back is to create a home environment that minimizes the opportunity of producing discomfort. A little thought and organization can greatly improve the way one feels. In turn, this decreases pain without sapping precious energy reserves.

How can this be accomplished? Consolidate and simplify household chores—cook for two meals at once, take breaks, and perform only simple tasks when energy levels are low. Arrange activities to decrease the times needed to walk up and down stairs. Avoid putting things that get a lot of use in high cupboards, and cabinets should have large handles for grasping. Rolling carts offer accessible, additional workspace. Use felt marker pens, which put less stress on the hands, and don't write for long periods of time. Of all the regular household activities, vacuuming is the worst. A vacuum cleaner's use aggravates back, shoulder, and arm discomfort and produces pain more often than any other appliance. Break up the activity. For starters, buy a lightweight vacuum cleaner and don't try to vacuum the whole house at once. When washing dishes, distribute body weight with one foot on a stepstool and try not to lean too far forward. Similarly, put one foot on a foot stool while ironing to reduce back strain. When washing windows, dusting, or scrubbing, find devices with longer, larger handles. If necessary, have somebody help carry in the groceries. Make your house more user friendly. If appropriate, put grab bars in the bathroom, change front door handles to levers, raise electrical outlets and phone jacks to a higher level, buy nonskid rugs, and use pull-out drawers or Lazy Susans.

Time and energy are too precious to squander—and this is one area where fibromyalgia patients have a lot of control.

AUTOMOBILES AND TRAVELING

It's important to get out and around, and most fibromyalgia patients travel in a car. Body mechanics in an automobile can make things better or worse. Bucket seats are more comfortable than bench seats. Make sure that the seat is adjustable and has armrests. The ideal vehicle for fibromyalgia patients should have an adequate headrest at the middle of the head for support, a climate control system, and automatic transmission. Mirrors should be plentiful, well placed, and easy to adjust. Don't recline, slouch, or sit too close to the steering column. For those with low back problems, buying a lumbar cushion or Sacro-Ease-like accessory may be useful.

While on vacation, take plenty of breaks from driving or sightseeing, find a flexible travel partner, and get a good night's sleep. Some fibromyalgia patients bring their own neck collars or pillows with them. Don't be shy about using special luggage racks, carts, or wheels. Don't let isolation creep into your life—go out, travel and enjoy!

HOW DO INFECTIONS INFLUENCE FIBROMYALGIA?

Most fibromyalgia patients have normal immune systems and don't get colds or other infections more frequently than other people. However, infections can aggravate fibromyalgia symptoms, and patients often take longer to recover. For example, when fibromyalgia patients develop bronchitis, persistent coughing frequently intensifies myofascial pain in the upper back. Fevers decrease stamina to a greater extent than in a healthy person. Viruses can lead to temporary relapses of fatigue syndromes. It's important to cope with these frustrations in a productive way. Some fibromyalgia patients need to pace themselves and take it a bit more slowly than usual for a little longer.

THE INFLUENCE OF EXERCISE AND REHABILITATION ON THE MIND AND BODY

Let's continue on the self-help road to improving fibromyalgia symptoms. Suppose we are eating healthy, well-balanced meals, are no longer smoking, have learned to pace ourselves, cope with changes in the weather, are sleeping well, and have reconfigured the house. At this point, how can the body be trained to reduce pain, stiffness, and fatigue? We will now explore how physical, mental, and complementary modalities allow fibromyalgia patients to feel better about their bodies and minds.

Therapeutic regimens that help the body and mind, whether physical therapy, yoga, acupuncture, or chiropractic methods, are all based on similar tenets of body mechanics:

1. Fibromyalgia patients will never improve unless they have good posture. Bad posture aggravates musculoskeletal pain and creates tight, stiff, sore muscles. Therefore, stretch, change positions, and have a good workstation that does not require too much leaning or reaching.
2. The way we get around is a demonstration of body mechanics. The fundamental principles of good body mechanics in fibromyalgia include using a broad base of support by distributing loads to stronger joints with a greater surface area, keeping things close to the body to provide leverage, minimizing reaching, and not putting too much pressure on the lower back (demonstrated in Fig. 13). Also, don't stay in the same position for a prolonged period of time.
3. Exercise is necessary. It improves our sense of well-being, strengthens muscles and bones, allows restful sleep, relieves stress, and releases serotonin and endorphins, which decreases pain and burns calories.
4. Don't be shy about using supports. Whether it be an armrest, special chair, brace, wall, railing, pillow, furniture, slings, pockets, or even another person's body, supports allow fibromyalgia patients to decrease the amount of weight or stress that would otherwise be applied to the body, producing discomfort or pain.
5. All activities should be conducive to relaxation and stress reduction, whether they be deep breathing, meditation, biofeedback, or guided imagery.

There is a surprisingly large number of ways these activities can be carried out. They are discussed in the next few sections.

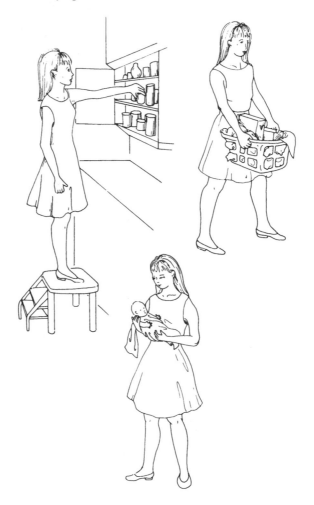

Fig. 13 *The basic principles of proper body mechanics that enhance well-being in fibromyalgia.*

PHYSICAL MODALITIES

The traditional methods for strengthening muscles, improving body mechanics and posture, and preventing damage are through exercise, physical therapy, and occupational therapy.

Why Does Exercise Hurt Me More?

Many patients with fibromyalgia were physically quite vigorous before they developed the syndrome. A common complaint is that when they tried to resume their activities, exercise only increased their exhaustion and pain. One survey showed that 83 percent of fibromyalgia patients do not exercise regularly and 80 percent are not considered physically fit. Some of the more common aggravating activities include heavy lifting or pulling. The CDC has even included "postexertion malaise" as a criterion for defining chronic fatigue syndrome. How can this paradox be explained?

As reviewed in Chapter 3, pain can result when muscles don't get enough oxygen. A consequence of changes in the ANS's signals is that this lack of oxygen and inefficient utilization of oxygen is further compounded by excessive constriction of blood vessels. In other words, when a fibromyalgia patient tries to exercise, a vicious cycle is unleashed. When blood vessels don't allow enough oxygen to be delivered to muscle tissue, even mild exercise produces microtrauma, or "angina," in muscles and pain. Further, microtrauma to the muscles can't be repaired at night since not enough growth hormone is released when we sleep poorly. In turn, these factors lead patients to avoid exercise in order to minimize discomfort. Over time, muscle atrophy, or wasting, and osteoporosis, or thinning of the bones, develop. This limits the patient's reserves and produces deconditioning so that even mild exertion results in profound fatigue.

What Is the Best Kind of Exercise for Fibromyalgia?

How can fibromyalgia patients overcome the vicious cycle of exercise-pain-fatigue-exercise-pain-fatigue? First, motivation to undertake a gradual, progressive course of increasing activity and exercise is important. Try walking as the initial activity. Walk for five minutes twice a day, increasing to 45 minutes. Take breaks or sit on a bench if this makes you feel fatigued or winded. Walking is the first step toward a general conditioning and toning program. It diminishes stiffness. Over time, it relieves muscle and vascular spasm and allows more oxygen to reach the tissues. If the weather is bad, walk in an indoor mall. Walking with a friend can take the mind off what's going on, and time passes more easily.

Gradually, other general conditioning programs such as swimming and bicycling can be added to the regimen. Swimming for 30 to 60 minutes three times a week is an excellent way to strengthen muscles and condition the body. The buoyancy of water moves joints through their full range of motion and strengthens muscles with less stress, as you move in ways that are difficult outside of water. Swimmers bear only 10 percent of their body weight. While swimming, increased chest expansion allows for deeper breathing and more oxygen to be taken in. Bicycling is an excellent activity that promotes general conditioning. Before buying a bicycle (stationary or otherwise), try it out and make sure the seat, handlebars, and amount of pedal resistance are comfortable.

Exercises are divided into several categories. In their simplest form, *isometric* exercises are useful in fibromyalgia. These routines allow patients to build muscle strength without moving, permitting a muscle to stretch until tension is felt. For example, the strap muscles in the neck can be strengthened by a cervical isometric program. If a patient pushes the forehead with moderate force against the hand placed against it and holds it for six seconds, the sustained muscle contraction (if repeated two times, twice a day along with other maneuvers as shown in Fig. 14) will strengthen the neck. This, in turn, protects patients against maneuvers, lurches, or sprains that increase upper back and lower neck strain. Along with isometric exercises, physical therapists frequently add *stretching* exercises to the regimen. Stretching does not allow jerking or bouncing around, decreases muscle tightness, prevents spasm and is performed together with deep-breathing exercises. A Pilates program is often very helpful. Fibromyalgia patients often have shallow, jerky breathing patterns; slow, deep, rhythmic breathing promotes energy and allows relaxation.

Over time, patients work their way up to *isotonic* exercises that start with low-impact aerobics, where at least one foot is on the floor and there is no jumping. In their most helpful form, after a warmup period these activities allow enough arm and body movement to increase the heart rate without producing a jarring sensation that often makes fibromyalgia worse. We encourage fibromyalgia patients not to place too much tension on tender areas and have found that pain is

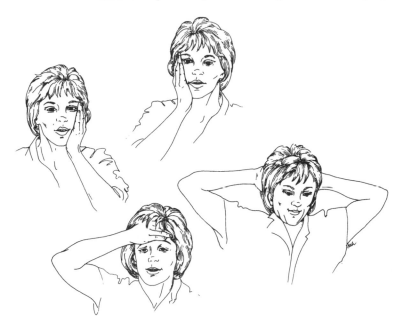

Fig. 14 *An example of strength-building isometric exercises. Performing these four cervical isometric maneuvers as sustained contractions for six seconds, twice a day, morning and evening, strengthens the sternocleidomastoid muscles and makes the neck less vulnerable to pain after injury or trauma.*

accentuated by weight lifting, rowing, jogging, or playing tennis, golf, or bowling early in the course of rehabilitation. Isotonic exercises are not for everybody and should be built up slowly. Make sure that a physician approves of the amount of exertion involved in an exercise program from a cardiovascular standpoint.

Aerobic exercises are designed to increase oxygen consumption by increasing the heart rate and are useful later on.

How Can a Physical Therapist Help Fibromyalgia?

Physical therapists are healthcare professionals who usually have had four to six years of formal education after high school. They help patients achieve physical conditioning by using several modalities, especially the sorts of exercises reviewed above. Some additional modalities are the following:

1. *Massage* allows deep muscles to relax, loosens tight muscles, relieves pain and spasm, improves circulation, and decreases stress. Massages should be gentle so as not to aggravate fibromyalgia symptoms. The Alexander Technique emphasizes posture and movement along with massage, and the Feldenkreis Method incorporates massage with body-mind communication enhancements.

2. *Spray and stretch* is a technique by which a cool spray (ethyl chloride or fluorimethane) is applied to a painful area, numbing the nerves locally, and is followed by gentle stretching of the muscle underneath it, promoting relaxation.

3. *Heat* relaxes muscles and can be applied with the use of blankets, showers, waterbeds, hot tubs, lamps, microwave gelpacks, heating pads, or a hydroculator. Moist heat is usually more effective than dry heat. Therapists frequently use ultrasound to deliver deep heat to painful areas in a relaxing, rhythmic motion. These sound waves go to the muscles, tendons, and soft tissues. A variant of this technique is iontophoresis, in which medication such as xylocaine or a local steroid can be administered to painful areas. Temperatures above 90° F (such as in a jacuzzi or hot tub) should not be applied to any area of the body for longer than 15 minutes since the treatment can produce lightheadedness, dizziness, low blood pressure, or excessive fatigue.

4. *Ice* or *cold packs* treat injuries or strains less than 36 hours old by decreasing swelling. Approximately 15 percent of our fibromyalgia patients prefer cold to heat and benefit from ice massages. Icing an area for 10–15 minutes before vigorous activity (e.g., the shoulder before playing tennis or the shins prior to jogging) minimizes postexertional muscle pain in patients who are deconditioned.

5. *Electrical stimulation* delivers electrical impulses to nerves that, in turn block painful messages. A form of electronic acupuncture, this can be accomplished by a TENS unit, acuscope, neuroprobe, or muscle exerciser.

6. Although chiropractors and osteopaths are known for their *manipulation* techniques, physical therapists also use traction, manipulation, and myofascial release.

7. *Posture and gait training* involves watching how patients walk and "carry" themselves. After evaluating a patient's body mechanics, the therapist may recommend strengthening and range-of-motion exercises, or assistive devices such as splints, collars, or braces.

8. The choice of *footwear* used while exercising or for everyday use is important. For the latter, the least expensive and most comfortable daily shoe is a sneaker a half-size too big. For exercise, there should be no pressure on the sides or toe tips, heel counters should hold the heel firmly, and the shoe should be comfortable. Shoes with widened toe areas or Velcro straps rather than laces may be desirable.

9. Physical therapists often work with occupational therapists or counselors to assist patients with *relaxation techniques.* These include biofeedback, deep-breathing exercises, guided imagery, and meditation.

If you are getting physical therapy at a large institution, try to see the same therapist each time. Camaraderie and close working relationships are associated with better outcomes.

What Is an Occupational Therapist?

The term *occupational therapist* is very misleading. Vocational rehabilitation counselors, not occupational therapists, advise patients about what employment is best for them and arrange for appropriate coursework and training. Occupational therapists practice a discipline known as *ergonomics* in designing work tasks to fit the capabilities of the human body. They perform an ADL, or Activities of Daily Living Evaluation. Occupational therapists consider such questions as: How much energy do people waste performing various chores such as housework? Is there a better way to get into and out of a car, on and off a toilet seat, or into and out of a bathtub? Occupational therapists apply principles of energy conservation and joint protection in their evaluations. Many large companies have therapists on site to evaluate workstations, office furniture, computer screen levels, and distances. Is the office environment smoke free, aesthetically pleasing, and user friendly? Is there adaptive equipment such as a longer or thicker handle that decreases reaching, bending, or lifting? Is splinting or bracing useful? Occupational therapists are experts when it comes to using or designing special wheels, levers, lightweight objects, enlarged handles, or specialized convenience tools. In our opinion, these underutilized professionals are the unsung heroes responsible for a portion of the increased corporate productivity that the United States has enjoyed over the last 20 years.

When Is a Physical or Occupational Therapy Evaluation Useful?

In our experience, patients with mild fibromyalgia infrequently need a formal rehabilitation program. Many physical therapists have little training concerning the needs of fibromyalgia patients and should consider taking a course the Arthritis Foundation offers to be up-to-date. Unfortunately, only one-third of our patients tell us that physical therapy was very useful, one-third report that they felt fine for a few hours afterward before returning to their baseline condition, and one-third say that they felt worse because the program was too aggressive or hard on the soft tissues. In the hands of highly proficient physical and occupational therapists, chronically ill patients or those refractory to treatment can have dramatic responses to a well-designed, well-thought-out rehabilitation program.

We usually prescribe physical and occupational therapy in tandem with medication to our patients who perform moderate to severe activity. The ideal program consists of 12–16 45-minute sessions over 3–4 months, after which patients can exercise independently and do their own rehabilitation. Most insurance carriers will pay for 10–20 physical therapy sessions a year if the need is well documented. About 10 percent of our fibromyalgia patients, especially those with reflex sympathetic dystrophy, benefit from one or two years of physical therapy.

MENTAL MODALITIES

Mental health professionals have become increasingly interested in using their expertise and resources to help fibromyalgia patients. Most have some training, and many have degrees in medicine, psychology, counseling, or social work. Traditionally, these health professionals use a variety of techniques to decrease stress, enhance coping skills, diminish fatigue, build self-esteem, and improve interpersonal interactions. Patients must feel comfortable with their therapists, and there should be a minimum of distraction during therapy sessions.

Classical Psychotherapy

We refer 10–20 percent of our fibromyalgia patients to psychotherapists. Fibromyalgia patients who are the best candidates for classical psychotherapy are in touch with reality and capable of having stable relationships with people, looking at themselves realistically, and being introspective. They should be willing to accept personal responsibility, have no secondary gain from their symptoms, and be interested in learning how to deal with anxiety, anger, or frustration without "acting out." The goals of therapy sessions are to verbalize concerns, confront inappropriate behavior patterns, clarify or understand these patterns based on past experiences, and work through problems. Patients should be able to identify their fears and destructive thinking patterns. They should try not to blame or make broad judgments. The treating professional and patient must form a therapeutic alliance enabling patients to develop a constructive means for dealing with problems that are prolonging stress, fatigue, or pain.

Cognitive Therapy: A Newer Approach to "Brain Fatigue"

Cognitive therapy is a useful approach for patients with fibromyalgia who have difficulty learning, retaining, processing, recalling, finding words, focusing, concentrating, planning, or organizing. Cognitive dysfunction or impairment is usually intermittent and probably reflects spasm of blood vessels supplying oxygen to the brain as part of a dysfunctioning ANS (see Chapter 3). Most patients who report cognitive symptoms note that they are intermittent and of short duration. However, up to 10 percent of our patients have had to alter their lifestyles to accommodate cognitive symptoms. Cognitive behavioral interventions work to improve sleep, inactivity, and ANS awareness with the goal of increasing function, as well as decreasing fatigue, anxiety, and pain. Modalities used by therapists include simple relaxation, exercise, biofeedback, and spiritual counseling. Patients are educated about treating pain with nonprescription approaches.

Cognitive therapists usually are psychologists, occupational therapists, or speech therapists. They urge their clients to use memory aids such as placing project lists and Post-its around the house, decrease distractions, not to catastrophize, form mental pictures to assist with associations, and not to get frustrated when trying to find words. Bad moods, depression, and anxiety can have a negative influence on memory. Therapists show patients how to use cues, designate one spot at home as the repository of all knowledge, and write things down so that they will not forget. Having regular daily routines, using timers or alarm clocks, and having a regular filing system also are useful. Be frank about the problem; covering up brain fatigue only makes things worse.

Biofeedback and Stress Reduction Strategies

Biofeedback works with making normally unconscious bodily actions conscious and controlling them to achieve relaxation and pain relief. Relaxation decreases SNS activity, slows the heart rate, and improves oxygen delivery to the muscles and brain. In particular, fibromyalgia patients have a heightened awareness of their autonomic functions such as pulse, blood pressure, and muscle tone. Electrical monitors can record skin temperature, heart rate, brain waves, digestion, and electrical skin conductivity (which measures muscle tension and is termed *EMG biofeedback*). Although at first glance it may seem like hocus-pocus, study after study has shown that deep-breathing exercises, relaxation tapes, and visualizing pleasant environments (called *guided imagery)* promote endorphin release and decrease muscle tension, pain, and stress. *EEG biofeedback* blocks some types of brain waves and reinforces others to improve cognitive, perceptual, and sleeping skills. For example, a qEEG, or quantitative EEG can measure the frequencies of alpha (idling), beta (alert), theta (awake but drowsy), and delta (sleep) waves. Patients are trained to increase their beta waves. Stimulation with *cranial electrotherapy* can improve sleep and decrease pain. Biofeedback can be administered by physicians, physical therapists, occupational therapists, or psychologists and is usually covered by insurance if the need for it is well documented.

Several controlled studies have shown that *cognitive behavioral therapy* improves fibromyalgia. These programs combine education, cognitive behavioral intervention, stress reduction techniques, support for family members and spouses, and strategies to improve physical fitness and flexibility. Biofeedback incorporates meditation, as do other techniques. For example, *yoga* combines deep breathing, meditation, and specific postures that integrate mental, physical, and spiritual energies to enhance well-being. *Transcendental meditation* enables patients to focus on a single thought or object to create an inner calm that banishes stress. *T'ai chi* adds passive movements to achieve this result. Also, never underestimate the power of *prayer* along with quiet contemplation.

Does Acupuncture Work?

According to ancient Chinese tradition, yin and yang are complementary aspects of chi, an energizing life force energy. Chi flows in the body through meridians, or imaginary lines along which the principles of acupuncture are based. Fine-gauge, sterilized needles are inserted along these meridians to allow "energy paths" signaling the brain to heal pain. Used for over 2,500 years, acupuncture ideally should stimulate endorphin release and diminish pain in fibromyalgia tender points. In our experience, acupuncture is safe and inexpensive. TENS units and dry needling stimulate A-delta fibers that diminishes pain by promoting the release of endorphins. The use of electrical acupuncture (see the physical therapy section of this chapter) is not restricted to the traditional meridians in relieving tender point pain. Most rheumatologists find the results of traditional acupuncture to be modest at best in managing fibromyalgia, and published studies show mixed results.

HOW TO OVERCOME FIBROMYALGIA: WHY COPING IS DIFFICULT

When our patients are diagnosed with fibromyalgia, their initial reactions are generally "What?" At this point, we provide them with literature from fibromyalgia support groups and the Arthritis Foundation and explain what this condition means.

It's hard enough to get through the day when feeling unwell. In fibromyalgia, the sense of being unwell is manifested by fatigue, pain, spasm, poor sleeping, lack of stamina or endurance, and sometimes difficulty concentrating or focusing. Fibromyalgia patients frequently react to these sensations with specific attitudes, emotions, and other behavioral responses, including anxiety, anger, guilt, loss of self-esteem, depression, and fear.

You Look Great! How Could You Be Sick?

There are no physical markers of fibromyalgia that reveal the syndrome to others. Fibromyalgia patients have no deformities, don't have an X marked on their forehead, look healthy, and seem able to be active. While this is good for the patient in one sense, friends, employers, and loved ones often have difficulty believing that they have so many complaints. Therefore, it's important to be open and frank with those who care. You need to have their trust to help them understand the limitations imposed by fibromyalgia. Patients do not need to be coddled or treated like invalids; they crave and need understanding and respect. Tell those who care that with a few modifications and a little time, you can still be as productive and as much fun to be with as before.

Anxiety

Anxiety is present in up to 70 percent of patients with fibromyalgia at some point during the course of the syndrome. It can be manifested by shortness of breath, palpitations, dizziness, lightheadedness, sweaty palms, trembling, chest pains, nausea, hot flashes, and, in extreme cases, a sense of impending doom or panic. Anxiety, in turn, worsens fibromyalgia symptoms, which sometimes can be hard to differentiate from those of anxiety. Anxiety is distressing but, if confronted firmly, will pass. Examine the causes of anxiety, face them, and don't run away. Patients must learn to relax and master their minds and bodies. Practice deep breathing, try to create a comfortable environment, write, or listen to pleasant music. Find ways to get a sense of control, dissipate the tensions of the day, create a sense of well-being, and get a good night's sleep.

Loss of Self-Esteem

Fibromyalgia is a formidable syndrome that can lead to loss of self-esteem. Hurting and being tired all the time takes its toll. Some patients cannot meet educational or career goals, lose the ability to be self-supporting, cannot engage in community activities, or experience cognitive impairment and difficulty focusing. This may lead to unstable or failed relationships with family and friends, with consequent loss of self-esteem.

The first thing a fibromyalgia patient needs to be aware of is a self-esteem problem. How did this happen? What can be done about it? Several steps can improve self-esteem in a fibromyalgia patient. Achieving a sense of personal worth promotes self-confidence. Visualize being happy. Do things that are enjoyable or help others. Stop being negative. Develop affirmations: I am courageous; I have options; I am not a victim; I am learning to relax; I can solve it. Peer counseling is frequently helpful in this situation. Getting back one's self-esteem is one of the first steps toward overcoming fibromyalgia.

Anger

Patients who get upset because they are not feeling well aggravate their fibromyalgia by tightening their muscles, making relaxation impossible. There are several self-help steps to confronting anger. First, conduct a personal reality check. Is there anything actually wrong with the way things are going? Are your loved ones healthy and alive? How are things financially? Don't get upset over things beyond your control, such as traffic jams or long lines at the supermarket. Deal with life's stresses in nonconfrontational ways. When making phone calls that require being on hold for a while, watch television or listen to music while waiting. Don't run errands that might require standing in long lines if time is a problem. Don't blame people for causing your problems or illness. Anger can be energizing, but channel it positively. There are healthy ways to express bottled-up anger. Think of how to prevent getting angry and how to relieve anger when it builds. Keep a chart or diary to award accomplishments in dealing with problems. It will help create a sense of well-being.

Guilt and Shame

Guilt has no place in fibromyalgia and makes the syndrome worse. Try to recognize its destructive effects. Regretting past behavior or thinking that you are bad are attitudes to be avoided. Don't berate yourself for things that fibromyalgia does not allow you to do. Overly perfectionistic tendencies can lead to guilt, as can unrealistic goal setting. Don't agonize over decisions that may have had unintended outcomes. We are all human, and we all make mistakes. Propose a rational response for dealing with guilt and looking ahead. Guilt is self-defeating. Develop a positive attitude to modify thoughts and behavior.

Depression

Patients do not develop fibromyalgia because they are depressed, but they can be depressed because they do not feel well. This reactive depression manifests as loss of interest and pleasure in life's daily activities. Classically defined as "helplessness and hopelessness," depression leads to a feeling of worthlessness, loss of appetite (or occasionally overeating), altered sleep patterns, loss of self-esteem, inability to concentrate, guilt, complaints of fatigue, and loss of energy. Patients who are depressed have lower pain thresholds, lose interest in personal care and grooming, have trouble making decisions, and sometimes get into more accidents or arguments. Depression affects the body, moods, relationships, and physical activities.

In order to overcome depression, fibromyalgia patients must first recognize that it's a problem and express a desire to do something about it. Once an ounce of motivation is kindled, some of the techniques discussed in Chapter 19 and later on in this chapter can be used to fight off depression. Medications prescribed to manage depression are reviewed in the next two chapters.

Perfectionism

Many of our fibromyalgia patients are overachievers. Prior to becoming ill, they led very busy lives with personal, work, and societal commitments. A perfectionistic tendency is evident where every detail of each daily activity is comprehensively thought out and analyzed. This needs to be differentiated from a psychiatric disorder known as obsessive-compulsive behavior, which is not associated with fibromyalgia. When the symptoms of fibromyalgia manifest themselves, fatigue makes it difficult to accomplish all the patient is able to do, which in turn creates feelings of guilt and inadequacy when the patient cannot perform. This leads to fears of failure and rejection and difficulty handling criticism. Overachievers need to adjust, think innovatively, learn to budget their energy, and delegate responsibility. Don't get so bogged down in detail that the overall picture is lost. Let initial frustrations evolve into relaxation. Life is too precious to waste on details beyond our control!

Fear and Trauma

A minority of patients with fibromyalgia had something terrible happen to them in the past, which makes it harder to overcome pain, poor sleeping patterns, and spasm. They may have been victims of abuse, neglect, a natural disaster, war, poverty, or crime. Don't let others convince these patients that a single factor such as a virus, a specific diet, or a genetic tendency is solely responsible for the illness. Counseling is absolutely critical. Patients need to verbalize their traumas and the fears that go with them. They need to confront the facts of the situation and work out a way to put the past behind them so that their lives can go forward. This may require relocating to a safer environment, ending abusive relationships, or altering work styles. Only at this point can fibromyalgia be effectively overcome.

SOLUTIONS: HOW TO IMPROVE COPING SKILLS

Develop Positive Goals and Attitudes

Patients should treat the diagnosis of fibromyalgia as a challenge to their resourcefulness. They should set realistic goals and be proactive. List all the problems, from easiest to hardest to resolve. Write down the remedies for each symptom, sign, and problem, one at a time. Follow the results. Reprioritize goals. Try not to do annoying, recurrent tasks. Don't be drawn into a no-win situation. Set limits and learn to say no. Avoid negative people. Instead of thinking that "it's hopeless and will never get better" or "this treatment will make me worse," try developing the attitude that things will get better and medication will help. Discuss medications with a doctor and inquire as to how they assist self-improvement. Decide if individual or group counseling is something that might expedite more positive feelings.

It's important to do positive things by challenging one's financial, personal, and intellectual resources. Cultivate spirituality. Develop new interests and hobbies. Seek positive news and information. Improve communication skills. If you are courteous and say "please" and "thank you," others will be helpful and pleasant in return. Give affection to others, and it will be returned. Don't worry about tomorrow; focus on what can be done today. Be open to receiving help and verbalizing thoughts; don't keep them suppressed. Patients who set attitude changes as goals really do start to feel better about themselves.

How to Improve Coping

In order to cope with fibromyalgia, be flexible and learn to adapt to the illness. Life can be happy in spite of fibromyalgia. Learn to understand the concept of self-responsibility and accept it. Most patients work, despite feeling unwell, by accommodating the illness. Explain what fibromyalgia is to spouses, relatives, and friends. The importance of seeking help and avoiding isolation cannot be overemphasized.

Dealing with Stress

In Chapter 3, we reviewed how stress or trauma can bring on fibromyalgia and reviewed the biochemical pathways by which this occurs. A recent survey suggested that 63 percent of fibromyalgia patients feel that stress is a major factor in influencing their symptoms, signs, and disease course.

How can stress be decreased? First, remember that lessening stress increases energy. In the beginning, learn to relax. Find a quiet environment and a comfortable position. Whether it's listening to soft music, practicing meditation, guided imagery, deep abdominal breathing, hypnosis, thinking of or inhaling pleasant aromas (*aromatherapy*), t'ai chi, prayer, or biofeedback, we support whatever works. Next, learn to say no and communicate your concerns. It may be necessary to accept limitations and modify job descriptions and workstations to limit physical and emotional stress. Budget time to allow for periods of re-laxation. Learn to pace. Make a list of everything that is stressful and how these factors can be avoided or improved. Also, enjoy distractions. Have fun. Learn to laugh. Listen to comedy shows or tapes, read a good book, or take up gardening. Get a pet. Develop a hobby. Distractions make it easier to perform necessary or required activities that are less enjoyable. Finally, remember that stress can cause and aggravate fibromyalgia by releasing chemicals that aggravate or accelerate symptoms of pain and fatigue.

Develop a Positive Doctor-Patient Relationship

Whether they are seeing a mental health therapist, physical therapist, chiropractor, or physician, patients must be able to communicate with their healthcare professionals. Since only physicians can prescribe medication or hospitalize, their relationships with and feelings toward patients are extremely important. Here are a few tips on how to maximize the doctor-patient relationship.

Find a doctor who believes that fibromyalgia exists and is interested in helping these patients. Avoid unreasonable expectations. Does the doctor have a genuine interest in the patient as a person? Does the physician reinforce the patient's self-esteem, listen, or allow disagreements or questions? Does the patient feel comfortable asking questions or feel too rushed? Does the doctor talk in plain English? Most important, will the doctor be the patient's advocate? Can he or she write jury duty letters, allow handicap placards if needed, fill out disability forms, and defend the patient in a legal deposition?

In return for these considerations, be sensitive to the doctor's needs. Be organized and honest. If it's hard to explain a problem, write it down and restrict the note to one page. What makes the complaint better or worse? What's been tried in the past? Do not argue with the doctor. Be informative and reasonable. Don't expect an instant cure. Follow the suggested course of therapy to completion—a noncompliant patient cannot expect to improve fully. Doctor-patient relationships are important partnerships that can be quite fragile at times.

If a physician referral is needed, call the nearest medical school, county medical association, Arthritis Foundation, or fibromyalgia support group.

Marriage, Sexuality, and Family

Married or unmarried couples may wish to probe how their relationships interact with fibromyalgia and vice versa. Make sure that the partner knows what fibromyalgia is and how he or she can help the patient enjoy life. Open communication decreases resentment and resolves potential conflict. Be on the lookout for potential problems. Does the partner resent or attempt to control the fibromyalgia patient? Does he or she buffer upsetting information before telling the patient? Does the mate derive satisfaction from caring for a fibromyalgia patient? Does the mate feel neglected or unable to help?

A good sexual relationship is a source of pleasure, self-esteem, and relaxation, which also decreases stress. Fibromyalgia should not interfere physiologically with lovemaking. The uncommon exceptions include autonomically mediated dry vaginal walls (easily treated with lubricants) and significant spasm of vaginal muscles, often with a history of sexual or physical abuse. Occasionally, fibromyalgia medications can influence libido. Don't be afraid to ask a doctor about the potential side effects of medications before taking them. Enhancing intimacy while reducing stress should be a goal.

Relatives and friends should be helpful resources. Some fibromyalgia patients react to the disease by decreasing their social contacts and isolating themselves. "I'm too tired to do anything" or "I hurt too much to be away for more than a few hours" are warning signs of a developing problem. When patients complain of difficulty keeping up with household chores or meeting responsibilities to their children, relationships may become precarious. The sleep disorder of fibromyalgia can also alter intimacy. Develop a positive plan to be an active family member, taking limitations into account. Keep all communication channels open with family members. They should be a patient's biggest cheerleaders!

Sometimes, family strife can worsen fibromyalgia. If this is the case, identify the sources of stress that interfere with rehabilitation. Focus on the problems, develop means for dealing with them positively, and seek counseling if needed.

Community Resources and Self-Help Groups

In addition to a doctor, healthcare professional, family, mate, and friends, there are community resources. For example, many Arthritis

Foundation chapters conduct a "Fibromyalgia Self-Help Course." It educates patients about fibromyalgia and trains leaders, who in turn are able to lead rap groups or self-help sessions. They meet once a week for two to three hours over several weeks. Other fibromyalgia support organizations also have lists of patients and doctors in different areas of the country who are interested in the syndrome. Appendix 1 lists other agencies and organizations that assist fibromyalgia patients.

A self-help group usually consists of 5–20 members who meet on a regular basis (usually once a month) to share information and experiences. The group leader should allow time for questions and answers, give research and clinical updates, and permit presentations by healthcare professionals. The leader should be strong yet empathetic, not allow one person to dominate the sessions, and set a positive, constructive tone. Members develop friendships that often provide additional support systems.

Finally, we need to address the Internet. Fibromyalgia patients surfing the Internet will find three basic sources of information: legitimate research and summaries of clinical papers put together by fibromyalgia support organizations or medical society Web sites; entrepreneurs trying to sell dietary or medically unproven remedies; and chat rooms where information, personal experiences, and concerns are shared. Try to stick to the sites recommended by the Arthritis Foundation or fibromyalgia organizations. Don't try any unproven therapeutic approach unless you discuss it with a doctor.

Dealing with Fibromyalgia in Children and Adolescents

Fibromyalgia is extremely uncommon in children. As a result, they often feel alone. Ask them to explain their pain. Make sure it's not a growing pain or early juvenile rheumatoid arthritis. Is reflex sympathetic dystrophy part of the syndrome? If so, this mandates a comprehensive rehabilitation program.

At school, don't let teachers accuse the child of being lazy. Educate them about the syndrome. Make things easier for the child, but assign him or her chores. Have the child use a knapsack that balances weight properly. Allow and encourage the use of markers or felt-tipped pens, which make writing easier. Don't stigmatize the child. Talk to the physical education instructor. Use colorful splints if needed. Ask the child what he or she thinks will be helpful at school and at home. Children are often afraid to verbalize their concerns.

Adolescents with fibromyalgia may be noncompliant in taking medications that alter mood, behavior, or appearance. All too often, doctors are unaware of this. Teenage girls often mistake menstrual symptoms for those of fibromyalgia. Adolescents need a role model apart from the immediate family to help them through difficult times. Whether the teen turns to a relative, coach, teacher, or clergyman, encourage this type of interaction. Talk to school officials and teachers. Encourage participation in extracurricular activities that don't aggravate fibromyalgia and allow the development of self-esteem and self-respect. Wrestling is out, but the school newspaper or yearbook, certain exercise classes, French club, or drama club are possible.

Fibromyalgia and Pregnancy

To our surprise, every year a patient of ours undergoes a therapeutic abortion because she believes that pregnancy has made her fibromyalgia too painful or that she will not be able to care for the baby. Women with fibromyalgia have fewer pregnancies than individuals without the syndrome. Some patients have told me that it would be impossible to get by without their medication and that they worry about its effects on the unborn.

What really happens during pregnancy? Pregnancy can aggravate fibromyalgia, but this happens only 20–30 percent of the time. Problems are associated more with sleep deprivation, hormonal changes, breast enlargement producing myofascial discomfort, morning stiffness, leg cramps, and low back pain, especially during the last trimester. Fatigue also can be a major problem. Yet, most of our patients do rather well and view these problems as worthwhile inconveniences considering the fulfillment of having a child. Even though manufacturers cannot guarantee successful pregnancies if their drugs are used, and routinely place warnings in the Physicians Desk Reference (*PDR*), studies suggest that pregnant women can take acetaminophen (Tylenol), tricyclic antidepressants such as Elavil or Flexeril, and specific serotonin reuptake inhibitors such as Prozac in the usual doses without worrying.

Sometimes fibromyalgia flares after delivery, especially if it is associated with postpartum depression. If medication is needed, be prepared to stop breast-feeding early or do not breast-feed at all. This gives the doctor greater flexibility in recommending medication. Carry the baby in a way that straddles the weight so as not to produce too much myofascial tension. Have the spouse handle some nighttime feedings to minimize sleep disruption. If financially feasible, consider hiring someone to help with baby care and housework. Many communities have mommy's-helpers programs through churches or community centers. The temporary inconveniences caused by pregnancy should be viewed as minor nuisances on a road that ultimately yields tremendous dividends!

Fibromyalgia in the Elderly

Fibromyalgia rarely develops in older patients for the first time, but as patients with the syndrome age, their problems grow. In addition to all the considerations previously noted in this chapter, there are a few additional points that warrant discussion.

First, some of the concerns we expressed about social isolation, communication skills, and community interactions need to be emphasized in elderly people. Once older persons cut themselves off from social outlets and stay indoors, their fibromyalgia worsens and their ability to function independently is impaired. Make sure that your senior citizen friend, colleague, or relative remains a viable member of the community. Also, doctors tend to put elderly patients on more medication. Whether they help the heart, blood pressure, lung, prostate, or diabetes, many of these agents interfere with fibromyalgia preparations. Some can worsen sexual performance; others can cause depression, promote aching or fatigue, or interfere with the ability to get around by producing lightheadedness or dizziness. Ask a doctor how any newly prescribed drug will influence fibromyalgia or interact with other medications given for particular health problems.

Older individuals need less sleep but are more affected by sleep medications, which produce dizziness or mental clouding. The development of osteoarthritis and osteoporosis with age tends to blur the distinction between fibromyalgia and another musculoskeletal diagnosis. Work with the family, community, and doctor to make the golden years truly golden.

COPING: SUMMING UP

Fibromyalgia patients frequently express feelings of anger, guilt, anxiety, and depression, which also aggravate the disease. There are ways to channel these feelings constructively, improve coping, relieve stress, devise positive goals, and assume favorable attitudes to make things better. Develop strategies, priorities, and organization, along with a support system of family, friends, coworkers, and the community, to stand up to the challenge of fibromyalgia.

10
Medicines for Fibromyalgia

ARE ASPIRINS OR NSAIDS BENEFICIAL?

NSAIDs and aspirin block the actions of a chemical known as *prostaglandin* that is responsible for some of the pain and inflammation of arthritis. Most fibromyalgia patients are familiar with these preparations, which are listed in Table 11. Preparations such as Advil, Aleve, or Orudis KT are available without a prescription.

Although these drugs are not dramatically effective in managing fibromyalgia, placebo-controlled, double-blind trials have shown that ibuprofen (the active ingredient of Advil and Motrin) and naproxen (Naprosyn, Aleve, Naprelan) in combination with other fibromyalgia remedies decrease pain in patients with the syndrome. They also alleviate premenstrual syndrome complaints, joint aches, and headaches. Doctors managing fibromyalgia patients recommend that these agents be used in any of several ways. First, they may be used on an occasional as-needed basis for pain breakthroughs. In this instance, blood counts need to be checked once or twice a year. Second, an NSAID may be prescribed on an ongoing, regular basis. In this case, patients should visit their doctor every three to four months and have laboratory testing, including a blood count, and liver and kidney function screening. Third, pharmacists are now making NSAIDs as gels or salves (particularly diclofenac and ketoprofen) that can be applied to painful areas. Aspirin-containing preparations such as BENGAY have been available for some time.

NSAIDs and aspirin are not without side effects. Patients who take these agents on a regular basis may experience fluid retention, bloating, upset stomach, diarrhea, or constipation. Ongoing administration requires checking patients for gastrointestinal ulcers, liver and kidney function, and rashes. The newer generation of selective cox-2 blocking NSAIDs (e.g., celecoxib, rofecoxib) are probably safer than older agents by producing fewer gastrointestinal bleeds or ulcers. In 1998, in the United States, 3 percent of regular NSAID users annually had gastrointestinal bleeds, often necessitating hospitalization. The selective cox-2 blockers should decrease this risk by 50–90 percent.

WHY DO DOCTORS PRESCRIBE TRICYCLIC ANTIDEPRESSANTS AND OTHER SIMILAR ANTIDEPRESSANTS?

Tricyclic antidepressants (TCAs) have been available for more than 40 years and represent the old, reliable approach to managing fibromyalgia.

Table 11. *Major NSAIDs*

Salicylates
    Aspirin
    Sodium salicylates (Trilisate, Disalcid)
    Diflusinal (Dolobid)
    Magnesium salicylate (Magan, Doan's)
Selective Cox-2 blockers
    Celeboxib (Celebrex)
    Rofecoxib (Vioxx)
    Valdecoxib (Bextra)
Propionic acid derivatives
    Oxaprozin (Daypro)
    Naproxen (Naprosyn, Anaprox, Aleve)
    Flurbiprofen (Ansaid)
    Ibuprofen (Motrin, Advil, Mediprin, Nuprin)
    Ketoprofen (Orudis KT, Orudis, Oruvail)
    Fenoprofen (Nalfon)
Acetic acid derivatives
    Sulindac (Clinoril)
    Diclofenac (Voltaren, Cataflam, Arthrotec)
    Tolmetin (Tolectin)
    Indomethacin (Indocin)
Oxicams
    Piroxicam (Feldene)
    Meloxicam (Mobic)
Others
    Etodolac (Lodine)
    Ketrolac (Toradol)
    Nabumetone (Relafen)
    Meclofenamate (Meclomen, Ponstel)

In doses lower than those demonstrated to alleviate depression, TCAs have a variety of beneficial effects on the syndrome. First, they may increase the amount of delta wave sleep. Second, they improve the availability of serotonin to nerve cells. Third, they heighten the effect of endorphins, which decreases pain. Finally, they relax muscles. These actions are accomplished by the combined effect of increasing levels of serotonin, dopamine, and norepinephrine, acting as an antihistamine and decreasing parasympathetic ANS activity. TCAs are not addictive, have no narcotic effect, and only indirectly decrease pain.

Which Tricyclic Should Be Used?

Numerous TCA preparations are available to treat fibromyalgia, but it often takes several attempts before the right dose and preparation are found for that individual. The most commonly used TCAs are listed in Table 12. The most commonly used preparation is *amitriptyline hydrochloride* (Elavil or Endep). Elavil is available as a 10-, 25-, 50-, 75-, or 100-mg tablet. Practitioners treating depression prescribe at least 25 mg a day, and 50–150 mg a day is probably a more effective dose. However, as little as 10 mg can decrease pain, relax muscles, and promote restful sleep. Since Elavil takes two to three hours to work, we advise most of our patients to take it several hours before going to sleep. Elavil usually lasts for about eight hours once it starts to work. Hence, if it is taken right at bedtime, one can have a "hangover"—a drugged feeling persisting into the midmorning hours. The beneficial effects of Elavil may not be fully evident for three to six weeks. We tend to prescribe doses of 10–25 mg at night. Some patients are very sensitive to TCAs. In these instances, we prescribe *doxepin hydrochloride* (Sinequan or Adapin) since doses as low as 3 mg can be derived from the liquid suspension. Doxepin dosing is the same as with Elavil, but for unclear reasons, doses of over 25 mg tend to promote considerable weight gain; as a result, we usually start with Elavil.

Cyclobenzaprine (Flexeril) is not marketed for depression and is approved by the FDA as a muscle relaxant. Consequently, we use this agent for patients with prominent musculoskeletal problems and few, if any, psychological problems. Its prescription also eliminates the stigma attached to taking an antidepressant. In our experience, 10 mg of cyclobenzaprine is equivalent to 15–25 mg of doxepin, and its actions are quite similar. We often advise patients to cut the tablet in half or even in quarters. Controlled studies repeatedly have documented the effectiveness of doxepin and cyclobenzaprine in managing fibromyalgia.

Certain patients have slightly different needs. For example, when depression is prominent, we tend to use *nortriptyline hydrochloride* (Aventyl, Pamelor), *imipramine hydrochloride* (Tofranil, Janimine), or *desipramine hydrochloride* (Norpramin, Petrofane) in Elavil-like doses, but we usually prescribe at least 50 mg in the evening. Patients who have more of a sleep problem and less of a pain problem often

Table 12. *Medication families clearly effective in treating fibromyalgia*

Tricyclic and closely related antidepressant preparations (TCAs)
    Amitriptyline hydrochloride (Elavil, Endep)
    Imipramine hydrochloride (Janimine, Tofranil)
    Doxepin hydrochloride (Adapin, Sinequan)
    Nortriptyline hydrochloride (Aventyl, Pamelor)
    Desipramine hydrochloride (Norpramin, Petrofane)
    Trazodone hydrochloride (Desyrel)
    Cyclobenzaprine hydrochloride (Flexeril)
Specific serotonin reuptake inhibitors (SSRIs)
    Citalopram (Celexa, Lexapro)
    Fluoxetine hydrochloride (Prozac)
    Sertraline hydrochloride (Zoloft)
    Paroxetine hydrochloride (Paxil)
Combination TCA-SSRI preparations
    Venlafaxine hydrochloride (Effexor)
    Nefazodone (Serzone)
Analgesics
    Tramadol (Ultram, Ultracet)
Central α_2 inhibitors
    Tizanidine (Zanaflex)
Benzodiazepines and closely-related drugs
    Clonazepam (Klonopin)
    Diazepam (Valium)
    Chlordiazepoxide (Librium)
    Alprazolam (Xanax)

derive benefit from *trazodone hydrochloride* (Desyrel) in doses ranging from 50–200 mg at bedtime.

What Are the Side Effects of TCAs?

The toxicity of TCAs varies considerably. The way they are broken
down, or *metabolized*, varies as much as 50-fold among patients. The
most common side effect is drowsiness, although 10–15 percent of
patients have a "reverse reaction" and become energetic after taking
the medication. In these instances TCAs can be taken in the morning,
but the sensation may be unpleasant to some patients and we usually
stop the drug when this happens. Occasionally we might try another
TCA, but if the patient complains of agitation or twitching, this is usually a signal to switch to a different family of drugs. Although dry
mouth, blurred vision, constipation, low blood pressure, and palpitations are the most common side effects of TCAs, manufacturers list
several hundred rare reactions to these agents in the PDR. Many of
these side effects can be ameliorated by lowering the dose or switching to a different preparation. Weight gain, fluid retention, and bloating tend to occur in antidepressant doses but are uncommon in
fibromyalgia doses. Cyclobenzaprine and trazodone produce these
complications least often.

TCAs should be used very carefully, if at all, in young children
(under the age of 12), in patients who are pregnant or breast-feeding,
and in elderly people who might become confused in the middle of the
night. For instance, when older patients are dizzy, sleepy, and have
poor balance, they could fall and fracture an osteoporotic hip when
they get up to go to the bathroom.

Sometimes, the effects of TCAs wear off with time. "Drug holi-
days," or weeks without using them or temporarily switching to a different TCA, can restore their effectiveness.

How Much Medication Should a Patient Take
and for How Long?

As we've noted, fibromyalgia patients generally don't like to take
medicine, and few doctors will prescribe TCAs if patients think they

must be taken forever. In fact, this need not be. We usually reevaluate our patients one month after starting a TCA. If their responses are favorable, the TCA is continued in a full dose for three to six months. At that point, we usually taper the drug to every other night and ultimately advise the patient to use it as needed. In other words, when a good night's sleep is critical, when it's been a particularly stressful time, when premenstrual symptoms are present, or if the weather has changed, a few nights on a TCA can be helpful. We have found that several months on a TCA tends to reset one's "pain thermostat," or threshold, and long-term use of the drug is frequently not needed. A summary of several published studies suggests that TCAs alone lead to a significant improvement in one-third of fibromyalgia patients and some improvement in another third after six months of treatment.

What do we do if the patient feels only somewhat better or does not respond at all? The sections that follow review other options.

WHAT ABOUT SPECIFIC SEROTONIN REUPTAKE INHIBITORS?

Specific serotonin reuptake inhibitors (SSRIs) are the newer kids on the block. Available since the mid-1980s, these drugs have revolutionized our management of depression. The use of these agents in fibromyalgia is a two-edged sword. *When taken by themselves (without a TCA or benzodiazepine), SSRIs can potentially make fibromyalgia worse.* Why? By promoting the release of serotonin, SSRIs reduce fatigue and increase energy. This, in turn, can make it difficult to sleep at night, which may aggravate fibromyalgia. As a result, early studies using SSRIs in fibromyalgia produced negative results. It was not until these agents were tested in *combination* with TCAs that it became clear that SSRIs can provide greater improvement in fibromyalgia than TCAs alone.

SSRIs are used to manage the fatigue, anxiety, cognitive impairment, and depression associated with fibromyalgia and can modestly alleviate pain by promoting the release of endorphins. They usually become effective within two to three weeks. SSRIs are not habit-forming and contain no narcotics. Also, as with TCAs, very low doses are often therapeutic; these doses are much lower than those used for depression. Patients with fibromyalgia are often very sensitive to all types of medication.

Available agents include the SSRI prototype, *fluoxetine hydrochloride* (Prozac). Since Prozac is available in 10- and 20-mg doses, and as a liquid suspension that can deliver as little as a few milligrams, we tend to start our patients at 5–20 mg a day in the morning. Prozac is stronger than other SSRIs and produces more agitation, sweating, headache, nausea, and palpitations. SSRIs can also help anxiety disorders and are now FDA approved for obsessive-compulsive behavior. Some patients have reported weight gain (only 20 percent lose weight) and decreased libido while using Prozac; second-line agents may be helpful if these side effects occur.

Physicians also can prescribe three "kinder, gentler" Prozacs— *sertraline hydrochloride* (Zoloft), *citalopram* (Celexa, Lexapro) and *paroxetine hydrochloride* (Paxil)—particularly for those with milder disease or a greater tendency toward drug side effects. The usual doses are 50–200 mg a day for Zoloft and 10–60 mg a day for Paxil. Recently, two combination TCA-SSRIs have become available: *venlafaxine hydrochloride* (Effexor) and *nefazodone* (Serzone). Although these preparations are very effective for depression, their use can be confusing in fibromyalgia since their effects on sleep are highly variable and must be monitored carefully.

As with TCAs, we try to use SSRIs for only a few months and let the body's pain and energy thermostat reset itself. After several months, we have found that SSRIs can reduce cognitive dysfunction and fatigue without disrupting sleep patterns, and these agents often can be used without TCAs.

BENZODIAZEPINES: THEY WORK, BUT USE THEM WITH EXTREME CAUTION!

Benzodiazepines relieve fibromyalgia symptoms primarily by eliminating the abnormal brain waves that produce the alpha-delta sleep wave abnormality and by decreasing sleep myoclonus, or restless legs syndrome. Approved by the FDA for use in epilepsy, a condition characterized by abnormal electrical impulses in the brain, these agents clearly have a place in selected patients with fibromyalgia.

Additionally, benzodiazepines are tranquilizers that promote relaxation and unspasm muscles. Their action is mediated by increasing serotonin and inhibiting transmission of excitatory nerve impulses in the brain or spinal cord via increasing levels of the neurotransmitter termed *gamma aminobutyric acid (GABA)*. Double-blind, controlled studies have established their efficacy in treating the restless legs syndrome and anxiety associated with fibromyalgia. *However, benzodiazepines must be used very carefully because they may be addicting and in a small minority of patients cause a serious depression that lasts until the drug is stopped.*

The principal agent used in fibromyalgia is *clonazepam* (Klonopin). One of the best drugs for epilepsy, twitching, restless legs syndrome, or jerking sensations, Klonopin, when given for fibromyalgia in doses of 0.5–1.5 mg at bedtime, promotes restful sleep and relaxes the muscles. It does little if anything for pain. It is a long-acting drug and may produce a morning hangover. It is otherwise well tolerated, with few side effects, the most common being fatigue and diarrhea. The effects of Klonopin decrease with time and the drug can be addicting after as little as several weeks of use.

When should one use Klonopin? We prescribe it for patients who cannot tolerate TCAs or have a suboptimal response to a combination

Table 13. *Dr. Wallace's approach to fibromyalgia therapies*

1. Give the patient a firm diagnosis, provide education about the disease, review physical measures and lifestyle approaches.
2. For 50 percent of patients we also prescribe medication. We tell them to use intermittent NSAIDs and start a TCA.
   a. One-third have an excellent response to the TCA, and many stop taking it within 6 months or use it intermittently.
   b. One-third need ongoing therapy with a TCA, with or without the addition of an SSRI.
   c. One-third have no response to TCAs or SSRIs and need other approaches.
3. One-third of patients benefit from an SSRI added to a TCA. Half of this group can discontinue the SSRI within 6 months.
4. One-sixth of patients are given SSRI-TCA combinations with benzodiazepines. Nearly half of this group ultimately report substantial relief.
5. One-sixth of patients have severe, resistant fibromyalgia and require additional agressive measures and therapies. Ultram and Zanaflex are useful adjunctive interventions.

of TCAs and SSRIs. Additionally, we use Klonopin for restless legs syndrome and to relieve acute steroid withdrawal symptoms. However, we advise our patients to take the drug only for two weeks at first. If additional or continued use is needed, we often ask them to take it every other night so that its effects will not wear off and it cannot be habit-forming. About 10 percent of the time, our patients develop severe, sudden depression. If this occurs, we stop the drug over several days and the depression subsides within a few days. Benzodiazepines can be administered with TCAs or SSRIs, and the combination may be useful.

Other drugs in the benzodiazepine family may be helpful. The much-maligned *diazepam* (Valium) also can be addicting and can cause depression. However, we occasionally use it for severe muscle spasms, for patients who want a Klonopin-like drug at night that is shorter acting, and for the 10 percent of fibromyalgia patients who have balance disturbances or dizziness. Valium is the drug of choice for benign positional vertigo, a syndrome brought on when changing positions causes dizziness, which can be an autonomic symptom of fibromyalgia. *Chlordiazepoxide* (Librium) has similar actions. Controlled studies have shown that it is particularly helpful for preventing convulsions in acute alcohol withdrawal and in irritable bowel syndrome (functional bowel disease) as the Librium-containing preparation Librax. Approximately 10–30 percent of fibromyalgia patients have anxiety, which may warrant treatment with medication. A controlled study conducted by Jon Russell at the University of Texas at San Antonio clearly showed that *alprazolam* (Xanax), in doses of 0.5–1.5 mg a day, decreases fibromyalgia-associated anxiety. Xanax should never be stopped suddenly. When no longer needed, it can be tapered slowly over several weeks.

TIZANIDINE: A NEW MUSCLE RELAXING ALTERNATIVE

Tizanidine (Zanaflex) activates brain and nociceptive alpha-2 adrenergic receptors that control SNS discharges. By facilitating neurotransmission at two sites in the brain and one site peripherally, Zanaflex relaxes skeletal muscles. In controlled studies, it decreases neck pain secondary to whiplash, tension headaches, neuropathic pain, and fibromyalgia pain. In doses of 2–8 mg at bedtime, Zanaflex helps some fibromyalgia patients sleep better, though up to 15 percent can have nightmares. We have used Zanaflex alone or in combination with TCAs and SSRIs. Patients taking Zanaflex should have their liver function tests checked regularly.

TRAMADOL: THE FIRST SPECIFIC AGENT FOR FIBROMYALGIA PAIN

Tramadol (Ultram) is a mild analgesic that promotes serotonin and norepinephrine. It was the first drug given by mouth that specifically blocks NMDA pathway receptors. However, the dose required to block fibromyalgia pain is six to eight 50 mg tablets a day (two tablets at a time, three to four times a day). Some patients feel a bit dopey on these higher doses, but in a double-blind, placebo-controlled trial, clear-cut long-term benefits were found. Recently, Ultracet (37.5 mg of tramadol with acetaminophen) has been introduced and produces less nausea while being just as effective.

MEDICINES THAT WORK: SUMMING UP

We frequently encounter patients who are so grateful to finally have a diagnosis explaining their symptoms and signs that, once they have read about fibromyalgia, they tell us that they will learn to live with it. Indeed, if the physical and emotional measures reviewed earlier are accepted, as many as half of all fibromyalgia patients in a community practice do not need any ongoing medication. Many of our patients take an occasional Advil and Aleve for pain during the day or Flexeril at night when they are stressed out or hurt more than usual. Despite this, at least 50 percent of our fibromyalgia patients are started on at least a TCA. One-third of them have a spectacular response, and many are able to stop the drug after several months and thereafter use it only occasionally.

Another third require the addition of an SSRI or a benzodiazepine, which leads to some improvement. Another third (or one-sixth of all fibromyalgia patients) do not respond satisfactorily to any of these measures. Some of the preparations discussed in the following sections are then prescribed, and this subgroup of patients usually benefits from psychotherapy given as an adjunct to physical measures and medication. Tables 12 and 13 summarize these concepts.

LOCALIZED REMEDIES

Do Tender Point Injections Work?

One of the most commonly employed interventions in fibromyalgia is the *tender point injection.* Controlled studies have clearly demonstrated its usefulness in patients with myofascial pain syndrome. When a patient comes to our office and reports that a specific point—for example, in the upper back or neck area—hurts, we try to ascertain how severe this discomfort is in relation to their overall pain. If we are told that at least 30 percent (and preferably more than 50 percent) of their pain at the moment is from a specific tender area, this is an indication for a local injection. Patients who "hurt all over" rarely respond to tender point injections for more than a few days.

Once we have decided to give a local injection or injections (usually limiting the number of injections to three per visit, with visits spaced several weeks apart), what preparations are used? The drugs of choice always include a local pain deadener, or anesthetic, usually xylocaine, Novocaine, or marcaine. After the painful area is sprayed with a coolant anesthetic such as ethyl chloride or florimethane, the anesthetic in the shots usually works immediately. Sometimes a steroid is added to the anesthetic in the same syringe.

Not all doctors use steroids for tender point injections. However, the doses we use are very low, and systemic effects are uncommon. The recommended preparations include *triamcinolone* (Kenalog or Aristocort), which is the most useful but must be given carefully since it sometimes dissolves fat tissue around the injection site and leaves a "pit;" *betamethasone* (Celestone), which is quite effective but burns more than other brands; *methylprednisolone* (Depo-Medrol), which does not last as long as the others but is well tolerated; and *dexamethasone* (Decadron LA), which is mild and well tolerated. The full benefits of these injections are usually apparent within several days, although patients may complain of local pain, flushing, or tingling for the first one or two days. The physician has to be very careful when injecting the upper back areas. He or she usually grasps or "lifts up" an area of fat or fascia to avoid puncturing the lung, a temporarily painful condition known as a *pneumothorax*. Pneumothorax is the most critical complication of the procedure, although it is very rare. Local injections can be given as often as needed, but we have found them worthwhile only if they provide relief for at least several weeks. Figure 15 shows how a tender point injection is performed.

What About Botox Injections?

Botox is a form of botulinum toxin Type A, a bacterial-derived substance that relaxes muscles through inhibition of alpha motor neurons. Approved by the FDA for strabismus and blepharospasm (lazy eye and constant winking), in controlled studies Botox injections clearly help some headaches and decrease neck pain secondary to whiplash. Some investigators have noted that some patients have had several

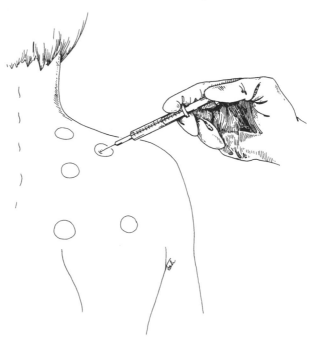

Fig. 15 *Example of a tender point injection.*

months of relief after injecting it into tender points. Injections into the pelvic musculature have improved chronic pelvic pain. Botox should only be used by practitioners experienced with its administration and can be quite expensive.

DO NERVE BLOCKS OR EPIDURALS WORK?

Nerve blocks are anesthetics and/or steroids injected into nerve tissues to relieve pain. Severe, localized, painful manifestations of reflex sympathetic dystrophy respond to nerve blocks, especially in the stellate ganglion area of the shoulder region.

Many patients with regional myofascial pain are incorrectly diagnosed as having herniated discs or arthritic disorders of the spine on the basis of abnormal X-rays, CT scans, or MRI scans. Unless an EMG with a nerve conduction study confirms that these abnormalities are producing physiologic changes, these X-ray or scanning results should be viewed with some skepticism. A recent study of healthy, asymptomatic people in their 40s who volunteered to have spinal MRI scans showed that 30 percent of them had significant abnormalities that rarely if ever caused symptoms. We have many fibromyalgia and myofascial pain syndrome patients who received epidural spinal nerve blocks for nonspecific radiographic abnormalities and localized symptoms that mimicked a disc disorder. The steroid in these epidural blocks often worsens the symptoms of fibromyalgia (see Chapter 13). Nerve blocks are usually prescribed only if there is clear evidence of a herniated disc or a degenerative process called *spinal stenosis.*

When Are Local Salves Used?

Topical gels, creams, ointments, and lotions have been used to treat local pain. Believe it or not, agents containing *capsaicin* (Zostrix, Dolorac) are cayenne pepper derivatives that locally deplete substance P (a pain neurotransmitter). These preparations frequently burn but are otherwise harmless and take a week or so to work. Give yourself the rheumatologist's version of the "Pepsi challenge!" Apply capsaicin for one week to one side of the body and see if it feels better than the other side. Other local preparations include *topical NSAIDs* and *aspirin.*

Topical anesthesia in the form of *EMLA* (eutectic mixtures of local anesthetics), *Lidoderm*, or *Tegaderm* block local pain for several hours by stabilizing nerve cell membranes.

MUSCLE RELAXANTS

In an effort to minimize muscle spasms and muscle pain, doctors prescribe a variety of muscle-relaxing drugs. However, unlike TCAs, tizanidine, or benzodiazepines, these agents have little or no effect on endorphins, pain threshold levels, pain perception, or emotional reactions, and only modest effects on sleep patterns. Nevertheless, in selected patients who have difficulty taking TCAs or who are not candidates for benzodiazepines, we sometimes prescribe muscle relaxants.

When muscle relaxants were first introduced, they were revolutionary and were frequently abused by patients and doctors. In the 1960s, use of the muscle relaxant *meprobamate* (Militown) was widespread, but the agent fell into disfavor when it was found to be highly addictive. A milder form of meprobamate, *carisoprodol* (Soma; Soma Compound contains aspirin), has become one of the most widely prescribed muscle relaxants in the United States. It acts on the nerves to relax muscles rather than on the muscles themselves. A double-blind, controlled trial suggested that Soma decreases pain, improves sleep quality, and increases the sense of well-being in fibromyalgia patients.

Preparations similar to Soma are also popular. All of these agents can produce fatigue and dull the senses a bit, and none of them should be used with alcohol. They are primarily prescribed for patients with acute low back pain or whiplash-induced spasm without fibromyalgia and are not intended for long-term use. An agent that unspasms muscles while promoting wakefulness is Norgesic Forte, a combination of aspirin, caffeine, and *orphenadrine citrate* (a muscle relaxant). Orphenadrine is also available without the aspirin and caffeine as Norflex. Other widely used preparations include *methocarbamol* (Rōbaxisal with aspirin, Robaxin without aspirin), *chloroxazone* (Parafon), and *metaxalone* (Skelaxin).

As noted in Chapter 3, magnesium plays a central role in muscle contraction. An interesting preparation containing *magnesium* and *malic acid* (available as Super Malate and Fibroplex, among other names) is available from health food stores. Controlled studies from England

and Texas in peer-reviewed journals have documented modest effects of this preparation on muscle spasm, fatigue, and pain in fibromyalgia. If patients take a dose larger than that recommended on the bottle (two very large pills three times a day), its effects become apparent within a week; side effects are uncommon. This combination may work as a result of interactions between magnesium and calcium channels within muscles and the generation of adenosine triphosphate (ATP), our cellular fuel. It occasionally induces diarrhea, drowsiness, lightheadedness, and dizziness at high doses.

Leg cramps are reported more commonly by fibromyalgia patients than by healthy people. They often respond to the administration of *quinine,* an old standby available since the 1600s.

PAIN KILLERS

Pain killers are analgesics that temporarily deaden the discomfort of fibromyalgia without reducing the underlying pain or its associated fatigue. Since higher and higher doses are needed after a while to maintain the same level of effectiveness, many pain killers are addicting. Narcotic preparations tend to be constipating, produce nausea, and reduce mental acuity. In one study, 36 percent of fibromyalgia patients required strong analgesics at some point in their treatment course, but fewer than 5 percent needed triplicate, or controlled narcotic-containing substances.

Drugs Marketed for Mild to Moderate Pain

The safest but least effective analgesic is *acetaminophen* (Tylenol). To protect the liver and kidney, patients should never take more than six tablets a day. NSAIDs and tramadol (Ultram) were discussed earlier in this chapter.

Drugs Marketed for Moderate to Severe Pain

We occasionally prescribe narcotic analgesics for short-term use (less than one week for acute flares) or for breakthrough pain (a few tablets a month). *Codeine* is available alone or in combination with either aspirin or acetaminophen but frequently causes nausea. *Propoxyphene* (Darvon) is similar to codeine in efficacy but is slightly weaker, and is also available in combination with aspirin (Darvon Compound) or acetaminophen (Darvocet-N). A few patients prefer the relatively nonaddicting *pentazocine* (Talwin NX or Talacen) for moderate pain.

Hydrocodone (Vicodin, with acetaminophen; or vicoprofen, with ibuprofen, Lortab) and *oxycodone* (Percodan, with aspirin, or Percocet, with acetaminophen) are very potent and highly addictive. Doctors should be on their guard if a patient requests Vicodin with Soma since this combination can produce a dangerous, addictive "high" and is sold as a street drug.

When Pain Becomes Unbearable

Stronger narcotics are available in many states as a triplicate prescription, whereby copies are sent to state or federal agencies for closer monitoring. Any physician who uses triplicate preparations should have some training in pain management techniques. Only a small minority of fibromyalgia patients ever require *morphine, hydromorphine* (Dilaudid), *levorphanol* (Levo-Dromoran), or *meperidine* (Demerol). Another opioid, *methadone,* may additionally block NMDA receptors. In pain management centers, these agents are also available as timed-release patches or in pumps for severe cases. In our experience, some fibromyalgia patients who progress this far also have severe psychiatric disorders or reflex sympathetic dystrophy. Despite their potency, morphine-like drugs often fail to relieve fibromyalgia pain. Opioid receptors become less responsive to actions of the NMDA pathway with time. Fibromyalgia patients with serious pain have the best outcome when they are managed at a multidisciplinary pain center employing the coordinated use of pain medications, nerve blocks, counseling, and physical rehabilitation techniques.

NERVE PAIN AND SPASM

Infrequently, patients with fibromyalgia report painful numbness, burning and tingling, or severe shooting spasms or jerks that do not respond to TCAs. Even though epilepsy is not associated with fibromyalgia, a group of agents used to manage seizures may be helpful in managing fibromyalgia complaints. These include *carbamezine* (Tegretol), *tiagabine* (Gabitril), *clonazepam* (Klonopin), *lamotrigine* (Lamictal), *phenytoin* (Dilantin), *valproic acid* (Depakote), and *gabapentin* (Neurontin). Tegretol blocks nerve responsiveness. Lamictal blocks sodium channels and stabilizes nerve membranes. Neurontin affects calcium channels and increases GABA levels, which slows down the central nervous system's nerve impulses. GABA also blocks the release of excitatory amino acids, which promote chronic pain. Patients using these agents should be followed on a regular basis, since the dosage and adjustments of these drugs should be supervised by a neurologist or another physician familiar with their uses and side effects, including monitoring of blood counts and liver tests.

Mexiletene (Mexitil) is a preparation known to be effective in managing irregular heartbeat. It is also helpful for diabetic neuropathy pain, and some of our fibromyalgia patients have had less nerve pain while taking it. *Baclofen* (Lioresal) relieves painful muscle spasms in some fibromyalgia patients by interacting with the GABA pathway (as do Valium-like drugs) to decrease spinal cord reflexes. It is usually prescribed for patients with multiple sclerosis, a condition not usually associated with fibromyalgia. A more toxic form of baclofen, *dantrolene* (Dantrium), should be avoided. Finally, a form of *L-dopa* (Sinemet 100/25) prescribed for Parkinson's disease (recognized by a shuffled walk and tremors) can successfully treat the jerks and twitches of restless legs syndrome that keep patients with fibromyalgia awake at night.

DRUGS THAT IMPROVE SLEEP

Despite using the measures discussed earlier, some patients still have difficulty sleeping. Occasionally, patients cannot take—or are unable to sleep in spite of taking—TCAs, or benzodiazepines. In a controlled study, the benzodiazepine-related agent *zolpidem* (Ambien) promoted sleep in fibromyalgia patients but did not relieve pain or morning stiffness. Few other sleep aids have been studied in fibromyalgia patients. Other benzodiazepines promote restful sleep but have little effect on the fibromyalgia. They include *florazepam* (Dalmane), *tenazepam* (Restoril), *oxazepam* (Serax), *zalepon* (Sonata), *quazepam* (Doral), and *estazolam* (ProSom). *Diphenhydramine* (Benadryl, Tylenol PM, Sleep-eze), *dimenhydrinate* (Dramamine), and *meclizine* (Bonine) are anti-histamines that induce drowsiness most of the time and have no demonstrated benefits in treating fibromyalgia. In a controlled trial, a nonbenzodiazepine not available in the United States, *zipiclone,* improved the sleep of fibromyalgia patients but did not reduce their morning stiff-ness, tenderness, or pain. Some sleep specialists have had success with an herb from *valerian root* (see Table 16). *Melatonin* is marketed as a food additive, but it is really a hormone made by the pineal gland of the brain. It regulates sleep cycles, increases growth hormone production, and increases acetylcholine release in brain cells. A 3–6-mg dose pro-motes a shallow sleep for four to six hours, but does not improve fibromyalgia pain. Fibromyalgia patients may have decreased melato-nin secretion. Barbiturates (e.g., Seconal, Nembutal, Placidyl) can be addictive, do not promote refreshing sleep, and are associated with sei-zures if suddenly withdrawn. They should be prescribed only by a sleep specialist, neurologist, or physician very familiar with their use. *Triazolam* (Halcion) should not be used since it has been associated with memory impairment. Restless leg syndrome interrupting sleep patterns respond to pramipexole (Mirapex), L-Dopa or Klonopin.

WHAT CAN YOU TAKE FOR A HEADACHE?

Headaches can be particularly disabling in fibromyalgia patients and are a major factor contributing to an impaired quality of life. Fibromyalgia-related headaches are either vascular, as in an autonomi-cally mediated headache, (e.g., migraine), or are caused by muscular tension. The latter results from osteoarthritic bone spurs in the neck or from myofascial tender points or muscle spasm in the back of the neck.

Vascular headaches in fibromyalgia patients may be treated acutely with NSAIDs; *ergot alkaloids* (e.g., Ergostat, dihydroergotamine, DHE-45, Migranol); epilepsy drugs, such as *valproic acid* (Depakote); or a Tylenol, sedative, and blood-constricting combination known as Midrin. Severe headaches can be relieved with agents that act on the serotonin receptors, such as *sumatriptan* (Imitrex), *zomitriptan* (Zomig), *riza-triptan* (Maxalt), *naratriptan* (Amerge), or, if necessary, with inject-able or oral narcotic analgesics such as *meperidine* (Demerol).

In addition to biofeedback and relaxation techniques, a variety of agents taken between headaches may prevent new attacks if headaches are persistent. These include *calcium channel blockers* (e.g., verapamil—Calan, Isoptin, Verelan); *tricyclic antidepressants,* such

Table 14. *Dr. Wallace's approach to headache in fibromyalgia patients*

1. Is the headache continuous or does it come and go?
   a. If it is continuous, obtain an MRI scan of the brain and, if the pain is in the back of the head or neck, obtain cervical spine X-rays. Is the neurologic examination abnormal? A neurologic or neurosurgical referral may be warranted if a tumor, disc, subdural bleed, abscess, aneurysm, or vascular malformation is present.
   b. If the headache is intermittent, is it a migraine (related to vascular spasm), cluster or histamine headache (related to foods or environmental factors), muscular tension headache, premenstrual, or sinus infection? If it is in the back of the neck, is it due to arthritis of the spine or to cervical muscle spasm? Is high blood pressure present?
   c. What makes the headache better or worse? Migraines are usually on one side and worsen with light exposure. Muscular tension is often associated with generalized fibromyalgia flares, and pains in back of the head improve with muscle relaxants or traction.
2. The treatment of an intermittent headache depends on its source, but a few general principles apply.
   a. Try acetaminophen or an NSAID (e.g., Aleve or Advil).
   b. If (a) is needed regularly, consider using a pain killer-muscle relaxant combination for acute, severe headaches on an occasional basis. These agents include Midrin, Esgic, Fiorinal, and Fioricet.
   c. If the therapies in (b) are needed regularly, consider ergots if migraine is present (e.g., Ergostat, Cafergot, Migranal), treat fibromyalgia systemically if muscles are very tight (e.g., Flexeril), or add physical therapy with relaxation techniques or cervical traction if neck and upper back pain is present.
   d. For severe, acute headaches that do not respond to (a), (b), or (c), the prophylactic regiments listed in (e) should be prescribed. Consider using a serotonin receptor agent (e.g., Imitrex, Maxalt or Zomig) injections, a nasal inhaler, or nasal pills until they work. Narcotic pain killers or Demerol shots are rarely necessary.
   e. If headaches do not subside, consider therapies that prevent headaches such as a calcium-channel blocker (e.g., verapamil), TCA (amitriptyline [Elavil]) or a beta blocker (e.g., propranolol [Inderal], atenolol [Tenormin]). Refer to a neurologist to rule out less common causes of headaches or use specialized approaches.

as amitriptyline (Elavil) in doses of 50–100 mg at night; and *beta blockers,* such as *propranolol* (Inderal). None of these preparations treat acute headaches, but when used between headaches, they prevent the development of new ones and break a headache cycle.

Muscular tension headaches are treated with NSAIDs, the muscle relaxants mentioned above, and drugs known as Fiorinal or Esgic, which are combinations of aspirin or acetaminophen, a small amount of a barbiturate, and caffeine, with or without codeine. These agents are highly effective and also relieve vascular headaches. However, they are intended only for occasional use since rebound headaches may result from suddenly interrupting regular use of caffeine, aspirin, or barbiturate-containing preparations.

Pain shooting through the back of the head, or occipital headaches from tender points in the upper neck area, are treated with physical measures such as cervical traction, massage, and other relaxation techniques in addition to NSAIDs, muscle relaxants, and trigger point injections. Table 14 demonstrates how we approach headaches in fibromyalgia.

TREATING GUT RESPONSES: NONULCER DYSPEPSIA (HEARTBURN) AND IRRITABLE COLON

Symptoms of heartburn, "acid indigestion," or reflux and esophageal spasm can be alleviated with dietary considerations (lactose restriction, more bulk) several types of agents, including *antacids* (such as Maalox or Mylanta, which are weak but inexpensive), *sulcrafates* (ulcer buffers such as Carafate, which is mildly helpful), or *H2 antagonists* (cimetidine [Tagamet], famotadine [Pepcid], nizatidine [Axid], ranitidine [Zantac]), which often give only partial relief. *Proton pump inhibitors* (e.g., omeprazole [Prilosec], esomeprazole [Nexium], lansoprazole [Prevacid]) are more effective in decreasing acid production and are generally meant for short-term or intermittent use. Lastly, *prokinetic agents* (e.g., metoclopramide [Reglan], erythromycin suspension) improve gut motility and decrease reflux. Make sure that your doctor tests for *Helicobacter pylori*, a common bacterial infection that can cause ulcers. There also are anecdotal suggestions that Tagamet boosts the immune system by activating B lymphocytes.

Abdominal pain, spasm, distention, bloating, and cramping are present in 30–40 percent of fibromyalgia patients. The dietary measures reviewed in Chapter 9 are helpful, but about half of these patients have severe enough symptoms to benefit, at least intermittently, from a variety of *antispasmodic* preparations that relax muscles in the intestine. These preparations include *dicyclomine* (Bentyl), the Librium derivative Librax, *tegaserod* (Zelnorm), *alosetron* (Lotronex), *hyoscyamine* (Levsin, Levbid), peppermint oil, serotonin receptor blockers (e.g., Zofran) and even *amitriptyline* (Elavil). A combination of a mild barbiturate and a muscle relaxant (Donnatal) taken at night decreases abdominal spasms and promotes restful sleep. Magnesium-containing preparations may relieve muscle spasms as well as constipation.

MEDICATIONS THAT HELP TO MANAGE DEPRESSION AND ANXIETY

Depression is associated with a lower pain threshold (see Chapter 3). The prevalence of depression or anxiety at any given time in fibromyalgia patients is a little under 20 percent and is over 50 percent during the course of the disorder. In our experience, 10–15 percent of fibromyalgia patients reach the point where they benefit from therapies other than TCAs, SSRIs, or benzodiazepines.

Several other families of drugs manage depression but have little, if any, influence on fibromyalgia. These include the *phenothiazines* (Thorazine, Mellaril, Prolixin, Stelazine, Risperdal, Haldol) for psychotic depression, *tricyclic-like* antidepressants (buproprion [Wellbutrin], amoxapine [Ascendin], maprotiline [Ludiomil], clomipramine [Anafranil, Mirtazapine, Remeron] for selected patients who have specific problems not ameliorated by TCAs or SSRIs, and *monoamine oxidase inhibitors* (phenelzine [Nardil], tranylcypromine [Parnate]) used for severe depression. The latter category has specific drug or food interactions, requires regular blood monitoring, and thus should be prescribed *only* in concert with treatment from a mental health professional.

Anxiety prevents fibromyalgia patients from enjoying life and functioning optimally. Controlled studies have shown that benzodiazepines such as *alprazolam* (Xanax) reduce this problem. However, if chronic anxiety is a problem, we prefer to prescribe nonaddictive drugs that are not sedating such as *buspirone* (Buspar). Buspar increases the availability of a selective serotonin receptor. Another useful agent is the t-acting benzodiazepine *lorazepam* (Ativan). Taken at bedtime, this drug is largely out of the system within four hours and helps anxious patients fall asleep.

CAN OTHER DRUGS HELP CHRONIC FATIGUE?

Of all the symptoms and signs reviewed in this chapter, patients most frequently ask for "something, anything" for fatigue. We usually use a TCA at first, since promoting restful sleep often alleviates daytime tiredness. Adding a serotonin promoter such as Prozac frequently provides an energy boost and improves symptoms of cognitive impairment.

For the remaining 15–20 percent of our patients who have significant fatigue in spite of TCA and/or SSRI therapy, we usually start with the mildest therapies and work our way up. First, we make sure that the patient is not anemic, does not have a low thyroid level, or does not have a high sedimentation rate, which would indicate systemic inflammation. There are numerous non-fibromyalgia causes of fatigue that have specific treatments.

Some practitioners swear by *vitamin B_{12}* injections, which in published studies help about 20 percent of patients and are harmless. At least one study showed that patients with chronic fatigue syndrome have decreased spinal fluid levels of vitamin B_{12}, and another study demonstrated increased spinal fluid levels of a closely related chemical, homocystine. Other physicians prescribe *thyroid* even if the thyroid blood level is normal. We generally discourage this since excessive or unnecessary thyroid administration can produce a rapid heart rate and anxiety and lead to premature osteoporosis. When the patient is overweight, some doctors have tried *diet pills* (phentermine, subutramine [Meridia], over-the-counter caffeine preparations). While these agents are mild stimulants, they also can produce anxiety and palpitations. The effects of dietary suppressants frequently wear off within a few weeks to months and are not a long-term solution.

WHAT CAN BE DONE FOR COGNITIVE IMPAIRMENT WITH OR WITHOUT FATIGUE?

Recent studies have suggested that a hormone produced by the adrenal gland, *dehydroepiandrosteone* (*DHEA*), may reduce cognitive impairment, but its mechanism of action is not clear. This agent is available from compounding pharmacies and health food stores as a food supplement and is not regulated by the FDA. We start at doses of 25–50 mg a day and sometimes go as high as 200 mg a day.

Severe cognitive dysfunction unresponsive to SSRIs may warrant a neurologic evaluation, which may include a type of brain imaging known as *SPECT scanning.* If not enough oxygen is getting to specific regions of the brain, milder amphetamine-like drugs such as *pemoline* (Cylert) are sometimes prescribed. Several published case reports have suggested that the extremely expensive calcium channel blocker *nimodopine* (Nimotop) dilates blood vessels and may improve thinking by driving more oxygen to the brain. We also have had some success with a form of counseling known as *cognitive therapy.*

Individuals in severe, vegetative states due to chronic fatigue, who cannot get out of bed for more than a few hours a day, should undergo a psychiatric evaluation and have their nutritional status evaluated. If a primary psychiatric diagnosis is ruled out, our group occasionally uses aggressive measures to help these patients function. *Fewer than 1 percent of fibromyalgia patients ever need to use any of the treatments reviewed in this paragraph.* They range from the attention deficit disorder (ADD) amphetamine *methylphenidate* (Ritalin) and *dextroamphetamine* (Dexedrine, Adderall) to *modafinil* (Provigil) the myasthenia gravis drug *pryridostigmine* (Mestinon), which promotes acetylcholine (and, indirectly, growth hormone) activity. Mestinon has been used to manage severe fatigue and cognitive impairment since the 1940s, and its efficacy was documented in early published clinical trials. However, in view of Mestinon's numerous side effects, a neurologist familiar with the drug's use should be consulted if a doctor does not have a lot of experience with it. A new mestinon-like agent, *donepezil* (Aricept), used to manage Alzheimer's syndrome, is being studied in a variety of cognitive dysfunction settings. *Dextromethorphan,* a chemical commonly part of cough medications (as DM, Delsym) shuts off NMDA receptors and impressively improves cognitive functioning in 10–20 percent of fibromyalgia patients. If the patient has autoantibodies, autoimmune activity, or any evidence of inflammation, the antimalarial drug *quinacrine* is available from compounding pharmacists and may be helpful.

A POTPOURRI OF POTENTIALLY
USEFUL REMEDIES

Fibromyalgia patients can have a variety of systemic complaints that require specific interventions. Doctors frequently treat symptomatic *mitral valve prolapse* with beta blockers such as atenolol (Tenormin) or propranolol (Inderal). *Female urethral syndrome* (irritable bladder) is managed with diazepam (Valium) or cyclobenzaprine (Flexeril) for a few nights when needed. If *interstitial cystitis* is present, dimethyl-sulfoxide (DMSO) instilled directly into the bladder desensitizes bladder nerve endings and relieves pain. An effective oral agent, pentosan polysulfate sodium (Elmiron), is also available. Individuals with *allergic* tendencies may be given antihistamines, antihistamine-phenothiazine combinations (Atarax, Vistaril), H2 blockers (Tagamet, Zantac), or short courses of corticosteroids as a pill, inhaler, or nasal spray. Newer-generation antihistamines that are relatively nonsedating and do not interfere with other drugs can be prescribed (fexofenadine [Allegra], cetirizine [Zyrtec], loratadine [Claritin]). NSAIDs and occasionally a muscle relaxant, vitamin B_6, or a diuretic for a few days until menses begin can alleviate *PMS* complaints. Patients with *autonomic dysfunction* often respond poorly to treatment, but serious neurally mediated hypotension can be improved with fludrocortisone (Florinef) or midrodrine by increasing blood volume or constricting blood vessels, respectively. We treat autonomic symptoms of burning and tingling with TCAs. Sometimes, agents that affect different parts of the ANS, such as the SNS beta blocker propranolol (Inderal), or the alpha-adrenergic promoter, clonidine, are useful. *Dizziness* is usually a form of vertigo; it responds to antihistamines or benzodiazepines.

ADJUNCTIVE THERAPIES: SUMMING UP

Most fibromyalgia patients who consult a rheumatologist are started on an NSAID, TCA, SSRI, or benzodiazepine. About half of these patients have additional symptoms or signs, which may lead to the prescription of at least one of the agents reviewed in this chapter. Most of these preparations are used on an occasional or intermittent basis. Toxic or habituating drugs such as narcotic pain medications, barbiturates, or amphetamine derivatives should be prescribed rarely, and only by

physicians with special training or expertise in pain management, r
rology, or psychiatry. Table 15 lists the drugs reviewed in this chapt..

Table 15. *Some examples of adjunctive drugs used to manage
fibromyalgia-associated conditions*

1. **Local remedies**
   Trigger and tender point injections
   Nerve blocks
   Topicals containing aspirin or NSAIDs
   Topicals containing capsaicin or xylocaine
   Topical anesthetics (Botox*)
2. **Muscle relaxants that are not TCAs**
   Pure muscle relaxants (e.g., orphenadrine [Norgesic], carisoprodol [Soma])
   Magnesium-malic acid combinations
   Quinine
   Tizanidine (Zanaflex)
3. **Pain killers that are not TCAs or SSRIs**
   Nonnarcotic: acetaminophen (Tylenol), NSAIDs, tramadol (Ultram)
   Nontriplicate narcotic: derivatives with codeine, propoxyphene (Darvon),
     hydrocodone (Vicodin)
   Triplicate (controlled) narcotics: morphine, oxycodone (Percodan), meperidine
     (Demerol), narcotic patches and pumps*
4. **Agents for nerve pain and spasm**
   Anticonvulsant derivatives (e.g., clonazepam [Klonopin], carbamezine
     [Tegretol], phenytoin [Dilantin], valproic acid [Depakote], gabapentin
     [Neurontin])*
   Mexiletene*
   Baclofen*
   L-Dopa*
   Other benzodiazepines (e.g., diazepam [Valium])
5. **Sleep enhancers that are not TCAs (also help vertigo)**
   Benzodiazepines (e.g., tenazepam [Restoril], florazepam [Dalmane])
   Zolpidem (Ambien)
   Antihistamines (e.g., diphenhydramine [Benadryl])
   Melatonin
   Avoid: Barbiturates, triazolam (Halcion)
6. **Headache relievers**
   For acute headaches: NSAIDs, pain killers (see no. 3 above), combinations
     such as Fiorinal, Esgic, Midrin, ergots, sumatriptan (Imitrex)
   To prevent headaches: calcium channel blockers (e.g., verapamil), TCAs, beta
     blockers

(Continued)

Table 15. *Continued*

7. **Functional bowel and nonulcer dyspepsia**
   Antacids
   H2 blockers (e.g., cimetidine [Tagamet]) or sulcrafate (Carafate)
   Proton pump inhibitors (e.g., omeprazole [Prilosec])
   Prokinetic drugs (e.g., metoclopramide [Reglan])
   Antispasmodic agents (e.g., hyoscyamine [Levsin])
8. **Depression and anxiety therapies that are not TCAs or SSRIs**
   Psychotic depression: phenothiazines*
   TCA- or SSRI-related agents (e.g., bupropion [Wellbutrin], maprotilene
      [Ludiomil])
   Monoamine oxidase inhibitors (MAOIs)*
   Antianxiety benzodiazepines (e.g., alprazolam [Xanax], lorazepam [Ativan])
   Buspirone (Buspar)
9. **Chronic fatigue and cognitive impairment therapies that are not TCA or SSRI responsive**
   Vitamin B$_{12}$
   Stimulants: Caffeine and amphetamine preparations*
   Related to systemic pathology: thyroid, iron, anti-inflammatory drugs
   Dehydroepiandrosterone (DHEA)
   Pyridostigmine (Mestinon)*
   Calcium-channel blockers (e.g., Nimodopine-Nimotop)*
10. **Mitral valve prolapse**
    Beta blockers
11. **Irritable bladder or interstitial cystitis that is not TCA responsive**
    Benzodiazepines
    Dimethylsulfoxide (DMSO)
    Elmiron
12. **Premenstrual syndrome**
    NSAIDs, diuretics, analgesics
13. **Dysautonomia**
    Beta blockers
    Fludrocortisone (Florinef), midrodrine
    Clonidine (Catapres)
14. **Allergies and chemical sensitivities that are not TCA or SSRI responsive**
    Hydroxyzine (Atarax, Vistaril)
    H2 blockers (e.g., cimetidine [Tagamet])
    Nonsedating antihistamines (e.g., fexofenadine [Allegra])
    Steroid inhalers or nasal sprays
15. **Treatments for dryness**
    Humidifying drugs
    Pilocarpine derivates

*Should be prescribed by an expert familiar with their use and closely monitored.

BEHIND THE HYPE: UNPROVEN, EXPERIMENTAL, HERBAL, AND INNOVATIVE REMEDIES

Numerous antimicrobial agents, vaccines, hormones, food supplements, and "immune boosters" have been purported to help fibromyalgia. This section will critically review our experience and that reported in the peer-reviewed literature with some of these preparations.

Antibiotics and Related Therapies

Viral vaccines have been used by a few alternative therapy physicians, but only a few poorly documented letters in chronic fatigue newsletters claim success. Yeast, or candida, is a fungus. The use of *antiyeast* preparations in the form of antifungal antibiotics (e.g., Nystatin, fluconazole [Diflucan], ketoconazole [Nizoral]) should be based on positive cultures for candida, *not* on antibodies indicating prior exposure to the fungus. Controlled studies have shown that fibromyalgia and chronic fatigue syndrome symptoms are not ameliorated by these therapies. We never prescribe antiyeast medicine unless a positive culture is present. Many antifungal preparations have potential hematologic and liver toxicity and should be regularly monitored. Yeast overgrowth, if truly present, infrequently leads to increased gas, bloating, fatigue, depression, or poor sleep habits. Using acidophilus decreases yeast by promoting the growth of good bacteria.

Hormones

Hormones are chemicals made in one organ that travel through the blood to another organ, where they have a physiologic action. Systemic *steroids* often cause a flare of fibromyalgia. *Adrenal cortex* is a natural steroid made by the adrenal gland that is available without a prescription. In larger doses it acts like prednisone, which can aggravate fibromyalgia and result in dependency. Our group showed that *calcitonin,* a hormone made by the parathyroid gland, modestly reduces bone pain in fibromyalgia patients in high doses but has no effect on fatigue or muscle pain. A few patients have reported increased well-being with *bromocriptine* (Parlodel), an agent that prevents prolactin from stimulating breast milk secretion. *Oxytocin,* a hormone made by the hypothalamus that is released during labor, lactation, and orgasm might improve pain, sleep, anxiety, and depression. *Thymus gland* extracts are heavily promoted in Europe for their "rejuvenating" properties, none of which have been borne out in peer-reviewed controlled trials. *Growth hormone* may repair muscle microtrauma (see Chapter 3), but this expensive preparation has many other potentially toxic effects. *Colostrum,* a form of breast milk may increase growth hormone levels. *Pregnenolone* and natural progesterones may be useful in selected patients with cognitive impairment, moodiness, or fatigue.

Vitamins and Food Supplements

Vitamins and food supplements are generally safe, though totally unregulated. Testimonial claims, commission sales, and pseudoscientific tracts annually bring in hundreds of millions of dollars to resourceful entrepreneurs. For example, there is ample evidence that under the microscope *antioxidants* are capable of cleaning up oxygen-containing free radicals that damage cells. However, no antioxidant is absorbed by the gastrointestinal tract and gets into cells in sufficient quantities to have any meaningful antioxidant effect on the body. This has not stopped purveyors of food supplements and vitamins from promoting literally hundreds of harmless and useless concoctions as antioxidants that make one feel good and retard the aging process.

The roles of *chromium, mushrooms, garlic, potaba,* and *liver extracts* have never been specifically studied in fibromyalgia patients. A negative controlled trial has appeared regarding *selenium. Magnesium, malic acid, creatine* and *NADH* may increase the amount of ATP energy packets in muscles and promote serotonin release. Patients with a rare group of muscle disorders known as *mitochondrial myopathies* may respond partially to *coenzyme Q10,* and reports have appeared suggesting that it lessens symptoms of cognitive impairment and fatigue. These preparations are very popular in Japan, where over 300 formulations are available, but controlled studies are needed.

Combinations of *free fatty acids* and *primrose oil* may decrease coronary artery disease and improve circulation, but their effects on tissue oxygenation in fibromyalgia have not been adequately studied. The late Nobel laureate Linus Pauling was a powerful advocate of megadose *oral vitamin C* supplementation in preventing infections and promoting a sense of well-being. However, we know of no evidence that expensive intravenous infusions of vitamin C are improving anything except the treating practitioner's wealth.

A by-product of vitamin B_{12} from pigs, *kutapressin,* has a cadre of alternative care physicians who swear by weekly injections, even though the only published controlled trial showed that patients who received placebo had an equal reduction in fatigue.

Amino Acids, Serotonin, and Immune Boosters

Amino acids are the building blocks of proteins. *L-threonine* may alleviate restless legs syndrome. *L-tryptophan* promotes serotonin but is potentially dangerous. A precursor of L-tryptophan, 5-hydroxy-tryptophan, is available from compounding pharmacies, but a controlled trial found it to be ineffective.

Ironically, an expensive antinausea drug that blocks serotonin and substance P, *ondensatron* (Zofran), was shown in a recent study to be mildly effective in fibromyalgia. Other selective serotonin receptor blockers such as *ritanserin* and *tropistron* may be beneficial as well.

We still don't know what role, if any, the immune system plays in fibromyalgia. Even though some studies have characterized chronic fatigue syndrome as a state of too much immune activation, some practitioners advocate giving "immune-boosting" *gamma globulin* infusions to these patients. Intravenous gamma globulin infusions are very expensive ($5,000 per month) preparations that modulate immune responses. Their use is restricted by hospitals and insurance companies to patients with serious immune deficiencies and certain autoimmune or neurologic disorders. A controlled trial reported that patients with chronic fatigue syndrome who received gamma globulin felt better than those receiving placebo. Other controlled trials have failed to confirm this, and the original trial's methodology has been questioned. An immune booster, *dialyzable leukocyte extract,* did not demonstrate any benefits in a clinical trial.

Guaifenesin and Other Odds and Ends

A California internist has popularized a theory that fibromyalgia results from a defect in phosphate metabolism and its resulting effects on muscle. An extension of this hypothesis states that agents such as an expectorant found in cold medicines, guaifenesin, promote the excretion of uric acid (crystallized uric acid causes gout), which helps fibromyalgia. None of the numerous muscle studies reviewed in Chapter 4 lend any support to this line of thinking, and the theory has never been published in any peer-reviewed medical journal. In fact, Dr. Robert Bennett at the University of Oregon conducted a double-blind, placebo-controlled, prospective trial that conclusively proved that guaifenesin is not only useless in treating fibromyalgia, it does not even promote the excretion of uric acid!

Topical salves with anesthetic or anti-inflammatory properties, such as hyaluron, gold, aurum (a combination of aspirin, camphor, and menthol), or quotane, may be helpful but have not been adequately studied. Topical *ketamine*, derived from the general anesthetic, blocks NMDA receptors and reduces pain. However it is difficult to prepare, is poorly absorbed, and its effects are highly variable. We reported that *hyperbaric oxygen* may improve cognitive impairment in fibromyalgia. Even though a negative controlled study was published, some doctors believe that the antidepressant *S-adenosylmethionine* (SAMe) may stimulate the central nervous system and help fibromyalgia. A sleeping pill not available in the United States, *zopicline,* improves sleep in the disorder but does not reduce morning stiffness, tenderness, or pain. Another sleep-promoting agent, *antidiencephalon serum,* may have modest effects. A few case reports have suggested that fibromyalgia responds to *lithium,* a drug given for manic-depressive psychosis. *Low-level laser* therapy has been delivered to painful areas with variable results. *Cartilage components* such as glucosamines and chondroitin sulfate help degenerative osteoarthritis, but these claims have no theoretical relevance to fibromyalgia. One prominent chronic fatigue specialist gives his patients *nitroglycerin* under the tongue to see if temporarily improving blood flow to the brain will make any difference. Nitroglycerin frequently causes headaches. Intravenous *lidocaine* may temporarily relieve pain by blocking C-fiber discharge, sodium channels, and NMDA receptors. In a well-controlled study, 8 of 63 patients receiving the infusion had a greater than 50 percent decrease in serious pain. *Gammahydroxybutyrate* (GHB) is used by some athletes to diminish fatigue and pain.

WHAT ABOUT HERBAL REMEDIES AND HOMEOPATHY?

Seed plants that are processed and used as medicine are known as *herbs*. The use of herbs as medicine dates back thousands of years and was independently developed by hundreds of cultures throughout the world. The pharmaceutical industry, mainstream physicians, and particularly alternative-therapy physicians have studied and recommended herbal remedies for a variety of ailments. Though no botanical remedies specifically for fibromyalgia have been studied, one of my rheumatologist mentors, Dan Furst, M.D., and his wife, Elaine Furst, R.N., have put together a useful "Herb Chart," which has been updated in Table 16 for informational purposes. They have concluded that some botanicals can be helpful, others can be harmful, and still others have no effect. Botanicals can be fresh or dried herbs, fluid extracts, or standardized extracts. Samuel Hahnemann (1755–1843) was a physician who rebelled against the vigorous and often unsuccessful therapies promoted by his allopathic colleagues discussed at the beginning of this chapter. In response, he founded the discipline of *homeopathy*. Homeopaths administer extremely small doses of natural extracts from plants, animal products, and minerals, some of which are harmful in larger doses, in an effort to stimulate a safe chemical response or effect.

Several homeopathic remedies are promoted as being helpful for arthritis and musculoskeletal pain. A few have been subjected to small, controlled trials, with contradictory results—half of them validating modest benefits. In our opinion, these agents are generally harmless, but their benefits in fibromyalgia are unproven.

ARE IMMUNIZATIONS OR ALLERGY SHOTS SAFE?

Fibromyalgia patients frequently ask whether or not they can receive routine immunizations and allergy shots out of concern for their immune systems. Nothing has ever been published or reported in the peer-reviewed literature suggesting that individuals with fibromyalgia react differently to these injections than otherwise healthy people.

Table 16. *Botanicals (for antiarthritics, skin treatments, and gastrointestinal treatments)*

Herb	Claimed Uses	Active Ingredients	Potential Side Effects
Alfalfa	Antiarthritic	Nonprotein amino acid (L-canavanine) and some saponins	In large quantities, could produce pancytopenia (decreased white blood cell count, anemia) could reactivate systematic lupus erythematosus
Arnica	Analgesic, anti-inflammatory (external application)	Sesquiterpenoid lactones (helenalin, dihydrohelenalin)	May cause contact dermatitis; cannot be taken internally; causes toxic effects on the heart and increases blood pressure
Black cohosh	Antirheumatic, sore throat, uterine difficulties	Substances that bind to estrogen receptors of rat uteri; also, acetin, which causes some peripheral vasodilation	Information on toxicity is lacking; could cause uterine bleeding
Burdock	Treatment of skin conditions	Polyacetaline compounds that have bacteriostatic and fungicidal properties	Side effects may result from addition with belladonna
Butcher's broom	Improve venous circulation, anti-inflammatory	Steroidal saponins (not corticosteroids)	Unknown; self-medication for circulatory problem is dangerous
Calamus	Digestive aid, antispasmodic for dyspepsia	Unknown	Use only Type 1 (North American) calamus, which is free of carcinogens is asarone (may promote cancers)
Calendula (marigold)	Facilitate healing of wounds (lacerations)	Unknown	Unknown
Capsicum	Counterirritant used to treat chronic pain (herpes zoster, facial neuralgia, or surgical trauma)	Capsicin (proven analgesic in osteo-arthritis, used externally)	Use caution in application; avoid getting into eyes or other mucous membranes; remove from hands with vinegar
Chlorella	Helps FM in one study	Green algae	Unknown
Catnip	Digestive, sleep aid	Cis-trans-nepetalactone (attractive only to cats)	Unknown; does not mimic marijuana when smoked

(Continued)

Table 16. Botanicals (*Continued*)

Herb	Claimed Uses	Active Ingredients	Potential Side Effects
Chamomilles, yarrow	Aids digestion, anti-inflammatory, antispasmodic, anti-infective	Complex mixture of flavonoids, coumarins, *d*-bisabolol motricin and bisabololoxides A+B	Infrequent contact dermatitis and hypersensitivity reactions in susceptible people
Chickweed	Treatment of skin disorders, stomach and bowel problems	Vitamin C, various plant esters, acids, and alcohols	Unknown
Comfrey	General healing agent stomach ulcer treatment	Atlantoin, tannin, and mucilage, some vitamin B_{12}	Hepatotoxicity (liver); can lead to liver failure, especially when the root is eaten; also causes atropine poisoning due to mislabeling
Cranberry	Treatment of bladder infections	Antiadhesion factors (fructose and unknown polymeric compounds) prevent adhesion of bacteria to lining of bladder	Increased calories if used in large doses (12–32 ounces per day; as a treatment rather than as a preventative (3 ounces per day)
Dandelion	Digestive, laxative, diuretic	Taraxacin (digestive), vitamin A	Free of toxicity except for contact dermatitis in people allergic to it
Devil's claw	Antirheumatic	Har pagoside	None
DongQuai	Antispasmodic	Coumarin derivatives	Large amounts may cause photosensitivity and lead to dermatitis, possible bleeding
Echinacea (purple coneflower)	Wound healing (external), immune stimulant (internal)	Polysaccharides, cichoric acid, and components of the alkamide fraction	Can flare autoimmune disease, allergies are possible; be sure product is pure and not adulterated with prairie dock (can cause nausea, vomiting)
Evening primrose	Treatment of atopic eczema, breast tenderness, arthritis	*Cis*-gamma-linoleic acid (GLA) (some suggestive data)	No data; borage seed oil (20% as GLA) may be a substitute and does have toxic side effects (liver toxicity, carcinogen)

(*Continued*)

Table 16. Botanicals (*Continued*)

Herb	Claimed Uses	Active Ingredients	Potential Side Effects
Fennel	Calms stomach, promotes burping	*Trans*-anethole, fenchone, estragole, camphene, L-pinene	Do not use the volatile oil—causes skin reactions, vomiting, seizures, and respiratory problems; no side effects with use of seeds
Fenugreek	Calms stomach, demulcent	Unknown	None
Garlic	GI ailments, reduced blood pressure, prevents clots	Allin (sulphur-containing amino acid derivative), ajoene	Large doses are needed (uncooked, up to 4 grams of fresh garlic a day), which may result in GI upsets; can "thin" the blood (anticoagulant)
Gentian	Appetite stimulant	Glysocides and alkalids; increases bile secretion	May not be well tolerated by expectant mothers or people with high blood pressure (possibly increasing pressure)
Ginger	Motion sickness, indigestion		Flares gall bladder disease, can cause depression
Gingko biloba	Helps dementia	Antioxidant	Very well tolerated, interacts with blood thinners
Ginseng	Fatigue, cure-all, anti-stress agent	Triterpenoid saponins	Be sure the product is pure; some insomnia, diarrhea, and skin eruptions have been reported; possible immune stimulant, interacts with insulin and blood thinners
Glycyrrhea glabra (Licorice)	Gastritis, reflux, cough		Don't use with hypertension, kidney disease
Goldenseal	Digestive aid, treatment of genitourinary disorders	Alkaloids (hydrastine and berberine)	In huge doses, may cause uterine cramps
Honey	Sore throat, antiseptic, anti-infective, antiarthritic, sedative	Fructose, glucose, tanin	Do not give to children under 1 year of age; may cause botulism in infants

(*Continued*)

Table 16. *Botanicals (Continued)*

Herb	Claimed Uses	Active Ingredients	Potential Side Effects
Kava kava	Sleep, stress, anxiety		Yellowish nail discoloration, incoordination, interacts with blood thinner
Lovage	Diuretic, promotes burping	Lactone derivatives (phthalides)	Some photosensitivity with volatile oil of lovage
L-tryptophan	Sleep aid, antidepressant	Essential amino acid that increases chemical serotonin, leading to some sleepiness	Be sure product is pure; contaminants may cause a serious blood disorder and a scleroderma-like illness
Mistletoe	Stimulates smooth muscle (American); antispasmodic and calmative (European)	Phoratoxia and viscotoxin (depending on the plant species)	Berries are highly toxic, and the leaves may also cause cell death; in animals lowers blood pressure, weakens, constricts blood vessels
Nettle	Antiarthritic, antiasthmatic, diuretic, against BPH	Histamine, acetylcholine, 5-hydroxy-tryptamine	Skin irritation from the active ingredients
New Zealand green-lipped mussel	Antiarthritic	Amino acids, mucopolysaccharides	No toxicity or side effects except in those allergic to seafood
Passion flowers	Calmative, sedative	Unknown or disputed	None
Peppermint	Calms stomach, promotes burping, antispasmodic	Free menthol and esters of menthol	Do not give to infants and young children, who may choke from the menthol
Pokeroot	Rheumatism, cure-all	Saponin mixture (phytolaccatoxin), mitogen, pokeweed mitogen (PWM)	Vomiting, blood cell abnormalities, hypotension, decreased respiration, gastritis
Rosemary	Antirheumatic, digestive, stimulant	Camphor, borneol, cineole, diosmin (a flavonoid pigment)	Large quantities of the volatile oil taken internally cause stomach, intestinal, and kidney irritation

(Continued)

Table 16. *Botanicals (Continued)*

Herb	Claimed Uses	Active Ingredients	Potential Side Effects
Rue	Antispasmodic, calmative	Quinoline alkaloids, coumarin derivatives	Skin blisters and photosensitivity following contact; gastic upsets when taken internally, may be an effective antispasmodic but is too toxic to be used
St. John's wort (Hypericum)	Antidepressant, anti-inflammatory, wound healing	10% tanin, xanthones, and flavonoids that act as monoamine oxidase inhibitors (antidepressants)	Photosensitivity dermatitis in those who take the herb for extended periods; Prozac-like, interacts with SSRIs, MAO inhibitors, digitalis
Sairei-to	Antiarthritic	12 herbs in combination	Diarrhea, abdominal pain, rash
Sassafras	Antispasmodic, antirheumatic	Safrole	Active ingredient is carcinogenic in rats and mice
Senna	Cathartic	Dianthrone glycosides (sennosides A+B)	Diarrhea, gastric, and intestinal irritation with large and/or habitual doses
Tea tree oil	Antiseptic (external application only)	Terpene hydrocarbons, oxygenated terpenes (terpinen-4-ol)	No side effects except skin irritation in sensitive individuals
Tumeric	Antiarthritic, ulcers	Unknown	Don't use with pregnancy, gall bladder disease
Valerian (garden heliotrope)	Tranquilizer, calmative	Unknown	None noted
Yucca	Antiarthritic	Saporins	None noted

Source: Compiled by Elaine E. Furst, R.N., and Daniel F. Furst, M.D. Modified from V. E. Taylor: *The Honest Herbalist*, 3 ed., Binghamton, NY: Haworth Press, 1993. pp. 336–351.

SUMMING UP

Few of the preparations mentioned in this chapter have proven efficacy in managing fibromyalgia. However, some of these agents are being studied in controlled trials and may prove useful in the future. Here's some friendly advice. Don't be talked into taking any preparation mentioned in this chapter without consulting a fibromyalgia specialist who is certified by a recognized specialty board. Let the buyer beware!

11
Work and Disability

Most of us have to work for a living. There are bills to pay and families to provide for. Since fibromyalgia patients do not usually look ill and on superficial examination appear strong, complaints of difficulty performing the job can be hard to believe. This chapter will review definitions as they apply to disability, impairments reported in fibromyalgia patients, and constructive approaches that allow individuals with the syndrome to work most effectively.

LET'S COME TO TERMS: WHAT IS DISABILITY?

The World Health Organization defines *disability* as a limitation of function that compromises the ability to perform an activity within a range considered normal. Efforts to manage work disabilities consider issues such as age, sex, level of education, psychological profile, past attainments, motivation, retraining prospects, and social support systems. Additionally, work disability issues take into account work-related self-esteem, motivation, stress, fatigue, personal value systems, and availability of financial compensation.

An *impairment* is an anatomic, physiologic, or psychological loss that leads to disability. Impairments include pain from work activities (e.g., heavy lifting), emotional stress (e.g., working in a complaint department), or muscle dysfunction (e.g., cerebral palsy). A *handicap* is a job limitation or something that cannot be done (e.g., deafness). Patients with a disability can be *permanently, totally disabled* and thus potentially eligible for Social Security Disability and Medicare health benefits. Other classifications include being *permanently, partially disabled,* whereby vocational rehabilitation, occupational therapy, and psychological or ergonomic evaluations can address impairments or handicaps to optimize employment retraining possibilities. *Temporary, partial disability* allows one to work with restrictions (e.g., no lifting more than ten pounds) while treatment is in progress. *Temporary, total disability* involves a leave of absence from employment while undergoing treatment so that one can return to work.

Subjective factors of disability include symptoms such as pain or fatigue, while objective factors of disability are physical signs such as a heart murmur or a swollen joint. One can be disabled from a *work category* and granted disability even if employment is ongoing in a different work category. Work categories are rated as sedentary, light work, light medium work, medium work, heavy work, or very heavy work, each defined by how much exertion is used over a time interval. Additional consideration is given to repetitive motions such as bending, squatting, walking up stairs, and squeezing, as well as environmental temperature or the operating of heavy equipment.

DO MOST FIBROMYALGIA PATIENTS WORK?

In the United States, up to 90 percent of fibromyalgia patients who wish to work are able to do so. Sixty percent of fibromyalgia patients are working full time. (The other 30 percent are housewives, househusbands, and retirees.) In a seven-university center study of 1,500 individuals with fibromyalgia, 25 percent had received disability payments at some time, and 15 percent received Social Security Disability (and Medicare) benefits. As noted before, studies from university medical centers include patients who have more severe problems and do not reflect the patient population seen in community-based rheumatology practices. Despite this, two-thirds of academic-based study patients related that they were able to work nearly all the time.

However, these statistics are deceiving and do not relate the problems fibromyalgia patients have had with employment. For example, in another survey, 30 percent of these patients had to change their jobs due to the disorder, and 30 percent modified their jobs in some way to accommodate their symptoms. All told, in the United States at any time, 6–15 percent of employed fibromyalgia patients are on some form of disability costing $10 billion a year in benefits and lost productivity. In nations with more generous disability systems such as Sweden, up to 25 percent of these patients are considered disabled.

WHY ARE SOME FIBROMYALGIA
PATIENTS DISABLED?

The most common reason fibromyalgia patients say they cannot work is severe pain. This creates many problems because pain is a subjective sensation that is hard for others to understand. After all, employers point out, other employees with pain are able to work. Additional factors that limit employment in fibromyalgia patients include poor cognitive functioning (inability to think clearly), fatigue, stress, and cold, damp work environments. Fibromyalgia patients complain of having decreased stamina or endurance and frequently have poor body mechanics. This limits their ability to undertake repetitive lifting, bending, or squatting, assume unnatural positions, or use excessive force. Using standardized test measurements in a study of light to medium jobs that required repetitive movements, fibromyalgia patients performed only 58.6 percent of the work done by healthy coworkers. This may be due to a decrease of up to one-third in muscle strength per unit for repetitive activities in patients with the syndrome. Interestingly, there is a discrepancy between perceived work ability and what is viewed on videos of work performance. Most fibromyalgia patients perform better than they think.

Another important factor relates to psychological makeup. Patients unable to deal with pain, low self-esteem, a strong feeling of helplessness, and low educational levels have a worse outlook. Do fibromyalgia patients malinger, or make up their symptoms for purposes of secondary (such as monetary) gain? Although offers of financial compensation are always attractive, several studies have shown that over 90 percent of the time, fibromyalgia does not stop working after litigation is settled. In Israel, where work disability is not recognized, trauma is associated with the same prevalence of postinjury fibromyalgia as in the United States. On the other hand, an epidemic of fibromyalgia-related "repetitive strain disorder" in the late 1980s in Australia was eliminated by minor changes in regulations.

WHAT RIGHTS DOES A FIBROMYALGIA
PATIENT HAVE?

The Americans with Disabilities Act protects individuals from job discrimination by requiring companies with more than 15 employees to make adjustments ("reasonable accommodations") for people with disabilities and chronic illnesses. These modifications include having an occupational therapist or ergonomic expert evaluate the work site. If fibromyalgia is brought on or aggravated by poor body mechanics or emotional stress caused at work, individuals are eligible for medical treatment, disability, and job retraining through the workers compensation system. Accommodations include part-time or half-day employment or a leave of absence. Most medium-sized and large companies have private disability policies. Although these approaches are all too often abused, their intent is to keep disabled people employed. If the disability is total and permanent, many individuals are eligible for Social Security benefits. Fibromyalgia, however, is not considered a disabling condition by the U.S. government. Therefore, the small number of patients with fibromyalgia who are totally, permanently disabled are usually granted Social Security benefits on the basis of related conditions such as chronic fatigue, pain, arthritis, or depression—all accepted disabilities under government rules.

HOW CAN TOTAL DISABILITY BE PREVENTED?

Despite all that has been related in this chapter almost 90 percent of fibromyalgia patients in the United States who wish to work can be employed in some capacity. In this section, we'll review strategies that enable patients to minimize pain and function as productively as possible.

1. **Find an agreeable environment.** Try to find a workplace that is quiet and smoke free, has clean air or is well ventilated, is adequately lit, heated, and has a comfortable noise level.

2. **Be up front and positive with your employer.** If fibromyalgia alters work performance or may require workstation or workplace modifications, let the employer know about the syndrome but do it in a positive way. Relate all the things you *can* do and how your productivity can be enhanced with minimal accommodations.

3. **Pace yourself.** Learn to manage time and prioritize job responsibilities and obligations. Make sure that a work day has several rest periods and a reasonable lunch break, which helps minimize fatigue. Focus your energy on what is important. Have a positive attitude and learn to laugh.

4. **Strategize and use coping skills.** Coworkers should be made aware of whatever adaptations are necessary for optimal productivity so that they will not view these as perks or become jealous. Learn to cope with the office environment—you cannot fire the boss. Don't get stressed out about what cannot be changed or about policies you do not control.

5. **Examine the workstation.** It is important to limit or avoid excessive lifting, reaching, twisting, standing, bending, overhead use of arms, and squatting. Consider using supportive braces or bands when engaging in these activities. Alternatively, follow employee manuals or physician or allied health professional (e.g., physical or occupational therapist) instructions if these motions are necessary for the job, since it's necessary to minimize harm from work trauma.

   Make sure your chair has a firm back and does not compress the circulation. Its height and back should be comfortable and at the right level for your computer keyboard. If the job requires heavy telephone use, consider using a speaker-phone or headset to minimize neck and upper back strain. Some individuals perform their work activities better if they wear back braces, rotate jobs, use rubber mats if prolonged standing is required, and are able to park closer to their office.

   Follow the recommendations in the computer manual regarding height, monitor angle, type of chair to be used, and screen glare. Keep arms parallel to hips, the hands above the keyboard and even or below the elbows, wrists straight, and fingers curved; special keyboards or soft pads may be helpful. When typing, arms should hang comfortably from the shoulders. The shoulder should be relaxed and not scrunched. An example is shown in Figure 16.

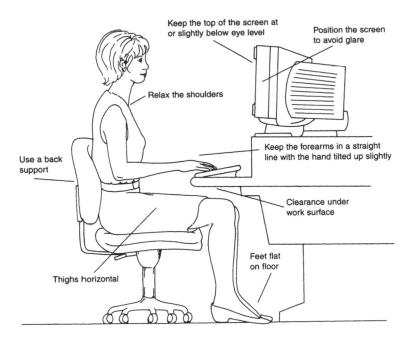

Keep the top of the screen at or slightly below eye level

Position the screen to avoid glare

Relax the shoulders

Keep the forearms in a straight line with the hand tilted up slightly

Use a back support

Clearance under work surface

Feet flat on floor

Thighs horizontal

Fig. 16 *An ergonomically correct workstation.*

6. **Help yourself.** Maintain correct posture to ease muscle strain, learn to relax, and keep physically conditioned. Take short work breaks to deep-breathe, relax, and stretch. Patients who have difficulty coping or who notice worsening pain shouldn't keep things to themselves. Call a doctor, mental health advisor, or physical therapist.

Unfortunately, our current disability system is insensitive to many of the considerations listed above and leads to more people not working than it should. This does not mean that the system should never compensate for fibromyalgia, but it needs improvement. The reason why 10 percent of people with fibromyalgia are permanently disabled is rarely the fault of the employer. The system needs to be changed so that these individuals receive treatment, and if necessary, Social Security disability as opposed to work-related disability.

SUMMING UP

The overwhelming majority of patients with fibromyalgia are able to work full time, but up to 40 percent may have to change jobs or make modifications in order to be productively employed. These individuals may take advantage of existing disability laws, protections, and medical resources to achieve this. The 5–10 percent of fibromyalgia patients who are totally, permanently disabled usually have severe problems with pain, fatigue, coping skills, or depression.

12
Prognosis and Future Directions

WHAT HAPPENS TO MYOFASCIAL PAIN SYNDROME?

When discomfort is limited to a specific region of the body and is not widespread, the outlook for long-term relief of pain is usually quite good. With local physical measures, injections, emotional support, and anti-inflammatory and analgesic medication, as well as instruction in proper body mechanics, over 75 percent of regional myofascial pain syndrome patients have substantial pain relief within two to three years. Unfortunately, there is little middle ground. For example, in an 18-year analysis of 53 patients with low back pain followed by musculoskeletal specialists, 25 percent ultimately developed fibromyalgia. Therefore, we believe that myofascial pain should not be shrugged off or given short shrift. A problem that is addressed early and effectively saves patients, health plans, and society money. Also ameliorated are the heartaches of patients and those close to them. Improved productivity promotes a feeling of relief, as well as a better quality of life.

WHAT HAPPENS TO FIBROMYALGIA?

The outcome of fibromyalgia depends on who sees the patient and calls the shots. For example, in one report that tracked family practitioners, internists, or other primary care physicians familiar with fibromyalgia's diagnosis and management, 24 percent of patients were in remission at two years and 47 percent no longer met the ACR criteria for the syndrome. This implies that early intervention by a knowledgeable community physician is the first line of therapy. Children with fibromyalgia also have a favorable outcome. In the largest study to date, symptoms resolved in 73 percent within two years of diagnosis.

The outlook in tertiary care settings is not as rosy. Once the symptoms and signs of the syndrome are serious enough to warrant referral to an academically oriented rheumatologist who is involved in fibromyalgia research, improvement is common but recovery rare. A summary of academic-based studies suggests that at three years, 90 percent of patients still have symptoms. They were rated as moderate to severe in 60 percent of the cases, and only 2 percent were cured. Among these patients, measures of pain, disability, function, fatigue, sleep, and psychological health change disappointingly little over the years. Those who fulfill the criteria for chronic fatigue syndrome tend to get better if they can trace their disease onset to an infection. Among this grouping, two-thirds are improved at two years. In our community rheumatology practice, we frequently find that most patients feel better after they are educated about the syndrome and treated. Many generally do well, but if the weather changes, a new emotionally stressful situation occurs, or physical trauma is sustained, relapse may occur. However, since these patients are connected to a rapid-response medical environment, long-term damage or disability can be prevented.

CAN A BAD OUTCOME BE PREDICTED?

Several investigators have tried to find unifying characteristics of patients who failed to respond to treatment. These individuals tended to have severe mood or behavioral disturbances, received less than 12 years of formal education, or were older than 40 when their symptoms began. In our experience, patients who are psychotic (those who carry the diagnosis of schizophrenia, bipolar disease, paranoia, or delusional disorder) or are not successfully treated for substance abuse do not improve.

WHAT CAN PATIENTS DO TO IMPROVE THEIR OUTLOOKS?

In the United States, too many health plans provide too much "tough love." As a result, fibromyalgia patients must be their own advocates. Patients with the syndrome should seek a practitioner who knows what fibromyalgia is, believes that it exists, and wants to help people with the disorder. If a health plan restricts access to this type of physician, patients should reiterate that nearly all health plans are required to provide the best possible care for specific problems. If this care is not available within a certain environment, the insurer must make accomodations to do the best for the subscriber's health and well-being. We're not talking about breaking the bank! A six-center survey of 538 chronic fibromyalgia patients treated in an academic setting (and, by definition, having more severe disease) had an average medical bill of $2,274 per year over a seven-year period. Fibromyalgia patients rarely benefit from surgery or hospitalization for their condition.

If fibromyalgia is identified early and managed appropriately, patients usually improve. Patients who know what fibromyalgia is and are motivated to improve their conditions fare better than passive individuals who get lost in the bureaucracy of our medical establishment. In our experience, it's harder for patients to improve (though not impossible) if therapy is delayed for more than five years. Individuals who are psychotic, demonstrate poor insight into their sources of psychosocial distress (if any), or who are addicted to drugs or alcohol, will not improve until their psychiatric and emotional problems are addressed first.

THE FUTURE HOLDS A LOT OF HOPE

The recognition of fibromyalgia by organized medicine as a distinct syndrome has had a salutary effect on research. As of this writing, 500 articles are now published yearly and $2 million is spent annually on research. All this attention and interest bodes well for more scientific breakthroughs in the field. What can fibromyalgia patients hope for over the next 20 years? We predict that 2–5 percent of the U.S. population has chronic neuromuscular pain with the systemic overlay mentioned above.

Over the next 20 years, the precise racial and ethnic backgrounds of these individuals will be identified, as well as the genes that influence the process. Additionally, environmental and occupational factors that cause or aggravate chronic neuromuscular pain will be clarified. Through coordinated strategies involving all forms of media, the public will become aware of what fibromyalgia is and what factors are associated with it. Increased awareness through an updated medical education curriculum will allow healthcare practitioners to intervene earlier to treat patients who develop fibromyalgia symptoms or signs after an injury or infection. This, in turn, will improve the prognosis and outcome. Better support systems will be available for individuals who require all forms of counseling or job retraining through the Arthritis Foundation and fibromyalgia support organizations.

BASIC RESEARCH ADVANCES

In the next decade, we predict that the body's pain pathways will be better demarcated and understood. Feedback loops and the source of what stimulates or suppresses certain "wires" or nerves will be elucidated. The roles of substance P, serotonin, the ANS, epinephrine, endorphin, dopamine, and other important chemicals that affect mood, pain perception, and transmission of information from one region to another will be better defined. For example, if we can block messages sent by excitatory amino acids (which amplify chronic pain but play no role in acute pain), a new class of drugs that specifically treats fibromyalgia pain can be formulated.

The nervous system does not work in a vacuum but involves interactions with hormones, the immune system, muscles, sleep, and stress factors. The biology of cytokines and other groups of chemicals that interrelate these components will be better understood. Along these lines, investigators will be able to answer several important questions in the next 20 years. Why are some behavior patterns associated with pain amplification but not others? Does muscle spasm result from a local reflex or does it come from signals within the spinal column? What does sleep have to do with growth hormone? Is there anything wrong with the immune systems of fibromyalgia patients? Why do reflexes within the ANS increase numbness, tingling, flushing, headaches, cramping, and burning rather than help people with fibromyalgia? How do viruses or other microbes cause chronic fatigue syndrome? What really goes on inside a local tender point?

FIBROMYALGIA THERAPIES: THE NEXT GENERATION

Current medications used to manage fibromyalgia will be improved. Newer, less toxic NSAIDs will be on the market in the next few years

Table 17. *Template, or categories for new drug development in fibromyalgia*

---

1. Chemical in the *ascending* pain tracts which could influence fibromyalgia
   NMDA blockers
   Nerve growth factor blockers
   Substance P blockers
   Ion channel modulators of sodium, calcium and magnesium
2. Chemicals in the *descending* pain tracts which could influence fibromyalgia
   Opiates
   Serotonin
   Dopamine
   Norepinephrine
   GABA
3. Chemicals that influence cerebral function subject to modification
   Cytokines
   Autonomic nervous system components
   Limbic kindling blockers
   Hormones
4. Anti-inflammatory approaches
5. Topical or local regimens which block limited or regional pain
6. Agents which modulate muscle metabolism
   Hormones
   Muscle relaxers
   Chemicals which influence blood flows to muscle or affect ATP

---

with the development of cyclooxygenase-2 antagonists. Safer and more specific TCAs (e.g., Elavil-like) and SSRI (e.g., Prozac-like) agents are on the horizon. Benzodiazepines (e.g., Klonopin-like) with less potential for inducing depression or addiction will be introduced. Vaccines against fibromyalgia-inducing infections may become available.

New classes of medicines will block substance P (e.g., Pregabalin); increase serotonin or adenosine A; release more endorphins; modulate calcium-magnesium in muscle channels or sodium channel blockers in cells; and block excitatory amino acids, nerve growth factor, and dynorphins. Agents that stabilize the ANS will be developed as our knowledge of cell signaling and cell surface receptors evolves. Biochemistry and neurochemistry advances will allow for the development and introduction of medications that act as kinin receptor antagonists, nitric oxide synthetase receptor antagonists, and tachykinin receptor antagonists and analogues of capsaicin. We may wish to augment or block certain cytokines. These approaches are summarized in Table 17. All of these preparations potentially are capable of decreasing pain and diminishing pain perception. Over the next 20–30 years, gene manipulation and control over apoptosis (programmed cell death) will challenge ethicists and scientists as we become capable of fundamentally manipulating our genes, cells, and progeny—thus, perhaps, greatly reducing the properties and production of pain.

Fibromyalgia patients should not give up hope. We've come so far in the last decade. Now, new exciting challenges are just beginning!

Appendix 1
Fibromyalgia Resource Materials

Many resources are available to fibromyalgia patients. In our previous effort, we listed numerous books and resources with addresses and telephone numbers. These listings became obsolete within a short time as new editions of books came out and nonprofit organizations changed their addresses and telephone numbers. The current information age allows this section to be much shorter. It will serve to guide the reader interested in learning more about fibromyalgia which listings in our opinion are the most helpful, and thus allow them to search the name or topic as a key word or person listing on the Internet.

WHAT OTHER BOOKS CAN I READ ABOUT FIBROMYALGIA?

The best books on fibromyalgia are written by musculoskeletal specialists (e.g., rheumatologists, physical medicine) who have treated patients with the syndrome and endorse concepts that pass scientific muster as documented by adequately controlled clinical trials, practice guidelines by medical societies, or in medical textbooks.

The following individuals or organizations have put forth such efforts:

> Arthritis Foundation
> Dr. Bernard Rubin
> Dr. I. Jon Russell
> Dr. Donald Goldenberg
> Dr. Mark Pellegrino
> Dr. Jay Goldstein
> Dr. Stanley Pillemer
> Dr. Harris McIlwain
> Dr. Roland Staud

WHAT ARE THE BEST VIDEOS AND BROCHURES THAT HELP US UNDERSTAND FIBROMYALGIA?

Similarly, pamphlets and videos are always being revised and can now be downloaded off the Internet. The following individuals or organizations have produced outstanding pamphlets and videos:

Beth Edinger
Dr I. Jon Russell
Jeanne Melvin
Fibromyalgia Aware magazine
Fibromyalgia Network
Fibromyalgia Alliance
National Fibromyalgia Association
Dr. Sharon Clark
Dr. Robert Bennett

I HAVE A MEDICAL BACKGROUND. HOW CAN I KEEP UP WITH DEVELOPMENTS IN THE FIELD?

The *Journal of Musculoskeletal Pain* and *Pain* publish more peer-reviewed fibromyalgia articles than any other journal. Some of the best work in the field appears in the *Journal of Rheumatology, Scandinavian Journal of Rheumatology,* and *Arthritis and Rheumatism.* Join the Fibromyalgia Network, Fibromyalgia Alliance and subscribe to their newsletter.

WHAT ORGANIZATIONS UNDERWRITE FIBROMYALGIA RESEARCH?

American College of Rheumatology
American Fibromyalgia Foundation
Arthritis Foundation
Fibromyalgia Alliance of America
American Fibromyalgia Syndrome Association
National Fibromyalgia Research Association
National Institute of Arthritis, Musculoskeletal and Skin
    Diseases (NIAMS)

ARE THERE OTHER ORGANIZATIONS THAT DEAL WITH FIBROMYALGIA-ASSOCIATED CONDITIONS?

Yes. There are hundreds. A few important ones are listed here.

American Academy of Physical Medicine and Rehabilitation
American Holistic Health Association
American Occupational Therapy Association
American Osteopathic Association
CFIDS Association of America (Chronic Fatigue and
  Immune Dysfunction Syndrome)
Lupus Foundation of America
National Headache Foundation
Scleroderma Foundation
Sjogren's Syndrome Foundation

WHO ARE THE EDITORS OF THE BEST RHEUMATOLOGY BOOKS USED BY DOCTORS?

Dr. John Klippel
Dr. William Koopman
Dr. William Kelley
Oxford Textbook of Rheumatology

Appendix 2
Glossary

acetaminophen   (Tylenol) a mild pain reliever occasionally useful in fibromyalgia.

acetylcholine   a neurotransmitter of the autonomic nervous system (see below) that induces dilation of blood vessels and slows down the gastrointestinal and urinary tracts.

acupuncture   traditional Chinese medicine therapy that reduces pain by inserting very fine needles just under the skin at points along "life force" pathways called meridians; in accupressure, manual pressure is applied instead of inserting needles.

acute   of short duration and coming on suddenly.

adenosine triphosphate (ATP)   molecule made in cells to store energy; probably decreased in fibromyalgia-affected muscles.

adrenal glands   small organs, located above the kidney, that produce many hormones, including corticosteroids and epinephrine.

adrenalin   see epinephrine.

aerobic   exercise designed to increase oxygen consumption.

affective spectrum disorder   a term used to consider irritable bowel, tension headache, irritable bladder, premenstrual tension, and fibromyalgia as being primarily of behavioral and secondarily of physiologic causation.

afferent nerves   nerves going from the periphery (e.g., skin, muscle) toward the spine.

alexithymia   long-standing personality disorder with generalized and localized complaints in individuals who cannot express underlying psychological conflicts.

allodynia   what happens when something that should not hurt causes pain; fibromyalgia is chronic, widespread allodynia.

alpha/delta sleep wave abnormality   delta waves make up most of slow wave, or nondream, sleep; alpha waves interrupting delta waves can produce movement or awakening, leading to unrefreshing sleep.

American College of Rheumatology (ACR)   a professional association of 5,000 American rheumatologists and 2,000 allied health professionals (the Association of Rheumatology Health Professionals).

analgesia   decreased perception of pain.

anemia   a condition resulting from a low red blood cell count.

ankylosing spondylitis   an inflammatory arthritis of the spine, sacroiliac, and sometimes peripheral joints; most patients have a positive HLA-B27 blood test.

anti-inflammatory   an agent that decreases inflammation.

antinuclear antibody (ANA)   proteins in the blood that react with the nuclei of cells; found in 96 percent of patients with lupus and in up to 10 percent of those with fibromyalgia.

artery   a blood vessel that transports blood from the heart to the tissues.

arthralgia   pain in a joint.

arthritis   inflammation of a joint.

Arthritis Foundation   a nonprofit national organization that provides patient support and funds research on musculoskeletal disorders.

aspirin   an anti-inflammatory drug with pain-killing properties.

autonomic nervous system (ANS)   part of the peripheral nervous system and divided into sympathetic and parasympathetic components; regulates stress responses, sweat, urine, and bowel reflexes and determines if a blood vessel constricts or dilates, thereby affecting pulse and blood pressure.

B-cell   a white blood cell that makes antibodies.

benzodiazepine   a potentially addictive group of drugs, including Valium and Klonopin, that relaxes muscles, among other actions, by blocking GABA (see below).

biofeedback   a training technique enabling an individual to gain some voluntary control over autonomic body functions.

biopsy   removal of tissue for examination under the microscope.

body dysmorphic disorder   a condition of individuals engrossed with themselves who express excessive concern or fear over having a defect in appearance.

bradykinins   chemicals that mediate inflammation and dilate blood vessels.

bruxism   persistently grinding one's teeth.

bursa   a sac of synovial fluid between tendons, muscles, and bones that promotes easier movement.

candida hypersensitivity syndrome   a controversial condition based on theories that a toxin released by yeast is responsible for irritable bowel, fatigue, and a feeling of illness; candida is a type of yeast, or fungus.

capillaries   small blood vessels that connect arteries to veins.

carpal tunnel syndrome   compression of the median nerve as it traverses the palmar side of the wrist, producing shooting nerve pains in the first to fourth fingers.

cartilage   tissue material that covers bone.

causalgia   sustained burning pain, allodynia, and overreaction to stimuli associated with autonomic nervous system dysfunction; reflex sympathetic dystrophy is chronic, widespread causalgia.

Centers for Disease Control (CDC)   an agency of the federal government based in Atlanta that monitors, defines, and sets standards for managing epidemics, infections, new diseases, and certain types of blood tests.

central nervous system   nerve tissue in the brain and spinal cord.

chiropractic   a therapy involving manipulation of spine and joints to influence the body's nervous system and natural defense mechanisms.

chronic   persisting for a long period of time.

chronic fatigue immune dysfunction syndrome (CFIDS)   a controversial term for chronic fatigue syndrome implying a prominent role for immune abnormalities.

chronic fatigue syndrome (CFS)   unexplained fatigue lasting for more than six months associated with musculoskeletal and systemic symptoms. Most of these patients fulfill the criteria for fibromyalgia.

cognitive behavioral therapy   the use of biofeedback-related techniques to improve speech and memory.

cognitive dysfunction   difficulty focusing, remembering names or dates, performing numerical calculations, or articulating clearly.

collagen   structural protein found in bone, cartilage, and skin.

complete blood count (CBC) a blood test that measures the numbers of red blood cells, white blood cells, and platelets in the body.

computed tomography (CT) a method of imaging a region of the body using a specialized type of X-ray.

conversion reaction a form of hysteria whereby an emotion is transformed into a physical manifestation (e.g., a person with normal vision claiming "I can't see").

corticosteroid any anti-inflammatory hormone made by the adrenal gland's cortex, or center.

corticotropin-releasing hormone (CRH) a chemical made in the hypothalamus of the brain that ultimately leads to the release of steroids by the adrenal gland.

cortisone a synthetic corticosteroid.

costochondritis irritation of the tethering tissues connecting the sternum (breastbone) to the ribs, producing chest pains; also called Tietze's syndrome.

cytokines messenger chemicals of the immune system.

dehydroepiandrosterone (DHEA) a hormone made by the adrenal cortex and also by the testes with male hormone properties.

delta sleep a type of electrical wave found on a tracing of brain waves during nondream sleep.

depression helplessness and hopelessness leading to feelings of worthlessness, loss of appetite, alterations in sleep patterns, loss of self-esteem, inability to concentrate, complaints of fatigue, and loss of energy.

disability a limitation of function that compromises the ability to perform an activity within a range considered normal.

dorsal horn nerves inside the back of the spinal cord; runs from the brain to the waist area.

dorsal root ganglion nerve cell bodies in the peripheral nervous system that receive nociceptive inputs and transmit them to the spinal cord.

dynorphin an opiate that suppresses acute pain but perpetuates chronic pain.

dysautonomia abnormal function of the autonomic nervous system.

dysfunction partial, inadequate, or abnormal function of an organ tissue or system.

dysmenorrhea   painful periods.

edema   swelling of tissues, usually due to inflammation or fluid retention.

efferent nerves   nerves that go from the spinal cord to its periphery.

electroencephalogram (EEG)   a mapping of electrical activity within the brain.

electromyogram (EMG)   a map of electrical activity within muscles; usually combined with a *nerve conduction velocity* study, which assesses nerve damage or injury.

endorphin   chemical substance in the brain that acts as an opiate; relieves pain by raising the body's pain threshold.

enkephalin   similar to endorphin (see above).

enzyme   a protein that accelerates chemical reactions.

eosinophilia myalgic syndrome (EMS)   a scleroderma-like thickening of fascia (see below) associated with high levels of circulating eosinophils caused by a contaminant of L-tryptophan; many patients with EMS develop fibromyalgia.

eosinophilic fascitis   a form of EMS (see above) probably induced by excessive shunting of L-tryptophan from the serotonin (see below) pathway to an alternative pathway.

epidemiology   study of relationships between various factors that determine who gets a disorder and how many people have it.

epinephrine   or adrenalin, a "nerve hormone" produced in the adrenal gland that acts as a neurotransmitter and stimulates the sympathetic nervous system.

Epstein-Barr virus (EBV)   a herpesvirus producing a mononucleosis-like illness that can lead to chronic fatigue syndrome.

ergonomics   a discipline that studies the relationship between human factors, the design and operation of machines, behavior, and the physical environment.

erythrocyte sedimentation rate (ESR)   see sedimentation rate.

estrogen   female hormone produced by the ovaries.

exacerbation   reappearance of symptoms; a flare.

excitatory amino acids   such as glutamate and aspartate function as neurotransmitting chemicals in chronic pain; when they are blocked, fibromyalgia pain is relieved.

fascia   a layer of tissue between skin and muscle.

fatigue   feeling weary or sleepy; may lead to reduced efficiency of work, accomplishment, or concentration.

female urethral syndrome   irritable bladder; persistent urge to void without evidence of infection, obstruction, stricture, or inflammation.

fever   a temperature above 99.6° F.

fibromyalgia   chronic, widespread, amplified pain associated with fatigue, sleep disorder, tender points, and systemic symptoms.

fibrositis   an outdated term for fibromyalgia (see above); discarded since it implies inflammation, which is usually not present.

flare   reappearance of symptoms; another word for exacerbation.

gamma-aminobutyric acid (GABA)   an inhibitory neurotransmitter.

gate theory   blocking or regulating transmission of pain impulses in the dorsal horn of the spinal column.

gene   consisting of DNA, it is the basic unit of inherited information in our cells.

growth hormone   made by the pituitary gland, decreased levels interfere with repair of muscular microtrauma during sleep.

Gulf War syndrome   a fibromyalgia-like disorder among Gulf War (1991) veterans probably caused by taking a combination of medicines meant to protect them from chemical warfare.

handicap   a job limitation; something that cannot be done.

homeopathy   a discipline based on the idea that symptoms can be eliminated by taking infinitesimal amounts of substances that, in large amounts, would produce the same symptoms.

hormones   chemical messengers made by the body, including thyroid, steroids, insulin, estrogen, progesterone, and testosterone.

hyperalgesia   exaggerated response to a painful stimulus.

hypermobility   laxity of ligaments allowing one to assume positions or undertake movements difficult for a normal person to do.

hyperpathia   delayed or persistent pain from noxious stimuli.

hypochondriasis   excessive preoccupation with the fear of having a serious disease based on misinterpretation of one or more bodily symptoms or signs.

hypoglycemia   low blood sugar level.

hypothalamic-pituitary-adrenal (HPA) axis   the system by which a releasing hormone secreted by the hypothalamus induces the pituitary gland to secrete stimulating hormone, which, in turn, induces the adrenal glands to release steroid-related hormones.

hypothalamus   brain region producing chemicals that release hormones.

hypoxia   insufficient oxygen reaching a tissue, organ, or region of the body.

hysteria   see conversion reaction.

immunity   a body's defense against foreign substances.

impairment   an anatomic, physiologic, or psychological loss that leads to disability.

incidence   the rate at which a population develops a disorder.

inflammation   swelling, heat, and redness resulting from the infiltration of white blood cells into tissues.

insulin-like growth factor-1 (IGF-1)   a byproduct of growth hormone (formerly known as somatomedin C).

interferon   sugar-protein substances with antiviral activity that can produce cognitive impairment with aching.

interleukin   sugar-protein substances that are intercellular mediators of inflammation and the immune response.

interstitial cystitis   a chronic inflammatory condition of the bladder.

irritable bladder   see female urethral syndrome.

irritable bowel syndrome   symptoms of abdominal distention, bloating, mucus-containing stools, and irregular bowel habits without an obvious cause.

joint   the articulation between two bones.

leaky gut syndrome   a controversial entity based on the belief that an overload of poisons overwhelms the liver's ability to detoxify, making the intestinal lining more permeable.

ligament   a tether attaching bone to bone, giving them stability.

limbic system   a collection of brain structures that influences endocrine and autonomic systems and affects motivational and mood states.

livedo reticularis   a lace-like pattern of small veins and capillaries visible on the skin.

lupus   (also systemic lupus erythematosus [SLE]) an autoimmune multisystemic disease caused by abnormal immune regulation resulting in tissue damage.

Lyme disease   caused when a deer-borne tick infects people with a bacterium; it is frequently associated with fibromyalgia and fatigue syndromes.

lymphadenopathy   swollen, palpable lymph nodes.

lymphocyte   type of white blood cell that fights infection and mediates the immune response.

magnetic resonance imaging (MRI)   a picture of a body region derived from using magnets; involves no radiation.

malic acid   works with magnesium to generate energy in cells.

melatonin   a substance made by the pineal gland of the brain that promotes sleep.

migraine   a vascular headache.

mitral valve prolapse   a floppy heart valve that can produce palpitations.

multiple chemical sensitivity syndrome   a controversial condition suggesting that chemicals in the environment produce symptoms and signs at levels not thought to be harmful.

muscle   a primary tissue consisting of specialized contractile cells that give strength to the body.

myalgia   pain in the muscles.

myelinated fibers   a fat-protein sheath surrounding nerve fibers.

myoclonus   twitching of a muscle or a group of muscles.

myofascial pain   discomfort in the muscles and fascia.

myofascial pain syndrome   fibromyalgia-like pain limited to one region of the body; also known as regional myofascial pain.

narcotic   an opiate-derived substance that suppresses pain.

National Institutes of Health (NIH)   a federal government organization that funds medical research.

neurally mediated hypotension   low blood pressure due to autonomic dysfunction.

neurokinins   substances made by nerves having physiologic effects.

neuropathic   pathology produced by compression, damage, or destruction of a nerve.

neuropeptides   consist of short chemical sequences common to amino acids (a building block of protein) that have effects on one's perception of pain and can act as neurotransmitters.

neuroplasticity   adapting to one's environment by modifying nerve structure or function.

neurotransmitters chemical substances that transmit messages through nerves.

nerve conduction velocity (NCV) measures the rate of nerve transmission and is usually part of an electromyogram (see above).

nervous tissue transmits information from nerve cells, or neurons.

nerve growth factor a chemical necessary for the growth and repair of autonomic and sensory neurons; triggers the release of substance P.

nicotinamide adenine dinucleotide phosphate (NADP) required for the production of energy in cells.

NMDA (N-methyl-D-aspartate) receptor a neurotransmitter sensor or receptor different from opiates that interacts with excitatory amino acids (see above); blocking it decreases pain.

nociceptor a nerve that receives and transmits painful stimuli; nociception is the process that transmits stimuli from the periphery (skin, muscles, tissues) to the central nervous system.

nonrestorative sleep waking up feeling unrefreshed.

nonsteroidal anti-inflammatory drugs (NSAIDs) agents such as aspirin, ibuprofen, or naproxen that fight inflammation by blocking the actions of prostaglandin.

norepinephrine a "nerve hormone" produced in the adrenal gland that acts as a neurotransmitter and stimulates the autonomic nervous system.

obsessive-compulsive disorder (OCD) persistent ideas or impulses; can include performing repetitive acts or perfectionistic tendencies.

occupational therapy uses ergonomics in designing tasks to fit the capabilities of the human body.

opiates narcotics.

organic due to a physiologic dysfunction as opposed to a psychological disorder.

orthopedist a doctor who operates on the body's musculoskeletal structures.

osteoarthritis a degenerative disease of the joints related to destruction of or defects in cartilage.

osteopath a physician who is trained in performing specialized physical manipulative modalities.

osteoporosis   loss of calcium from normal bone creating thin bones at risk of fracture.

oxytocin   hormone made by the pituitary gland; induces pregnancy labor and regulates small vessel circulation.

overuse syndrome   pain in muscles, ligaments, tendons, or joints from excessive activity in an area of the body.

pain   an unpleasant sensation or emotional experience.

palindromic rheumatism   intermittent swelling or inflammation of joints.

palmar erythema   redness of the hands due to an autonomic reaction.

parasympathetic nervous system   a division of the autonomic nervous system that blocks acetylcholine.

paresthesia   a sensation of numbness, tingling, burning, or prickling anywhere in the body.

pathogenic   causing disease or abnormal reactions.

peripheral nervous system   nerves to and from the spinal cord that transmit sensation and motor reflexes.

physiatrist   a practitioner of physical medicine (see below).

physical medicine   a medical specialty concerned with the principles of musculoskeletal, cardiovascular, and neurologic rehabilitation.

physical therapist   allied health professional that assists patients with physical conditioning.

pituitary   a gland in the brain that assists in the production of hormones.

placebo   a pill or treatment that has no physiologic actions or effect; a "sugar pill."

plasma   the fluid portion of blood.

pleura   a sac lining the lung.

pleuritis   inflammation or irritation of the lining of the lung.

polymyalgia rheumatica   an autoimmune disease of the joints and muscles seen in older patients with high sedimentation rates who have aching in their shoulders, upper arms, hips, and upper legs.

polymyositis   an autoimmune, inflammatory disorder of muscles.

positron emission tomography (PET)   an imaging technique that measures the flow of a substance to tissues; requires a cyclotron to perform.

prednisone; prednisolone   synthetic steroids.

premenstrual syndrome (PMS)   the release of chemicals prior to menstruation, causing fluid retention, alterations in mood and behavior, and sometimes painful periods.

prevalence   the number of people who have a condition or disorder per unit of population.

primary fibromyalgia syndrome   fibromyalgia of unknown cause.

prolactin   a hormone that stimulates the secretion of breast milk.

prostaglandins   physiologically active substances present in many tissues.

protein   a collection of amino acids; antibodies are proteins.

psoriatic arthritis   inflammatory disease of the joints in patients with psoriasis.

psychogenic rheumatism   complaints of joint pain for purposes of secondary gain.

psychosomatic   when parts of the brain or mind influence functions of the body.

rapid eye movement sleep (REM)   the part of sleep in which we may dream.

Raynaud's disease   isolated Raynaud's phenomenon (see below); not part of any other disease.

Raynaud's phenomenon   discoloration of the hands or feet (which turn blue, white, or red), especially with stress or cold temperatures; a feature of many autoimmune diseases.

reactive hyperemia   increased blood flow to an area following prior interruption or compromise of circulation.

receptor   area on a cell that receives chemical stimulation to activate a particular function.

referred pain   perceived as coming from an area different from its actual origin.

reflex sympathetic dystrophy (RSD)   a type of fibromyalgia associated with sustained burning, pain, and swelling.

reflexology   a form of alternative medicine based on the theory that specific areas of the ears, hands, and feet correspond to organs, glands, and nerves.

regional myofascial syndrome   fibromyalgia pain limited to one region of the body; also known as *myofascial pain syndrome.*

reactive arthritis   inflammation of the joints, conjunctivitis, mouth ulcers, and a psoriasis-like rash in patients who have a positive HLA-B27 blood test.

remission   a quiet period free from symptoms but not necessarily representing a cure.

repetitive strain syndrome   when repetitive motions in a work environment produce strain or stress on an area of the body, as in carpal tunnel syndrome from excessive typing.

restless legs syndrome   legs that suddenly shoot out, lift, jerk, or go into spasm; if this occurs during sleep, it is called sleep myoclonus.

rheumatic diseases   any of 150 disorders affecting the immune or musculoskeletal systems.

rheumatoid arthritis   chronic disease of the joints marked by inflammatory changes in the joint-lining membranes, which may give positive results on tests of rheumatoid factor or antinuclear antibody.

rheumatologist   an internal medicine specialist who has completed at least a two-year fellowship studying rheumatic diseases (see above).

scleroderma   an autoimmune disease featuring rheumatoid-type inflammation, tight skin, and vascular problems (e.g., Raynaud's disease).

seasonal affective disorder   when light deprivation during winter months produces depression and fatigue.

sedimentation rate   test that measures the rate of fall of red blood cells in a column of blood; high rates indicate inflammation or infection.

selective serotonin reuptake inhibitor (SSRI)   a class of drugs such as Prozac that treat depression and pain by boosting serotonin levels.

serotonin   a chemical that aids sleep, reduces pain, and influences mood and appetite. Derived from tryptophan and stored in blood platelets.

serum   clear liquid portion of the blood after removal of clotting factors.

sicca syndrome   dry eyes; can be due to decreased sympathetic nervous system activity, medication, or Sjogren's syndrome (see below).

sick building syndrome   allergy and fibromyalgia-like symptoms complained of by more than one person with extreme sensitivity to environmental components in the same home or workplace.

sign   an abnormal finding on a physical examination.

silicone   a synthetic organopolymer used in liquid form in breast implants and in solid form in joint replacements and intravenous tubing.

siliconosis   controversial syndrome implying that leakage of silicone from breast implants is responsible for systemic symptoms.

single photon emission computed tomography (SPECT)   a less sophisticated PET scan (see above) that does not require a cyclotron; in fibromyalgia it can diagnose cognitive dysfunction by documenting insufficient oxygen reaching the brain.

Sjogren's syndrome   dry eyes, dry mouth, and arthritis observed in many autoimmune disorders or by itself (primary Sjogren's).

sleep myoclonus   restless legs syndrome (see above) that occurs during sleep.

slow wave sleep   a phase of sleep not associated with dreaming but with alpha waves on an electroencephalogram (see above).

soft tissue rheumatism   musculoskeletal complaints relating to tendons, muscles, bursa, ligaments, and fascial tissues; includes fibromyalgia.

somatization   conversion of anxiety and other psychological states into physical symptoms.

somatomedin C   a form of growth hormone; see IGF-1.

somatostatin   blocks growth hormone secretion.

somatotropin   growth hormone.

spasm   increased muscular tension or involuntary muscular contraction.

spinoreticular tract   a trail of nerves that conducts impulses to the brain that regulate the autonomic nervous system from the periphery.

spinothalamic tract   a trail of nerves that conveys impulses to the brain associated with touch, pain, and temperature.

steroids   shortened term for corticosteroids, which are anti-inflammatory hormones produced by the adrenal gland's cortex or synthetically.

substance P   a neurotransmitter chemical that increases pain perception.

sympathetic nervous system (SNS)   a branch of the autonomic nervous system that regulates the release of norepinephrine (see above).

symptom   a subjective complaint relating to a bodily function or sensation.

syndrome   a constellation of associated symptoms, signs, and laboratory findings.

synovitis   inflammation of the tissues lining a joint; synovium tissue that lines the joint.

systemic   pertaining to or affecting the body as a whole.

systemic lupus erythematosus   see lupus.

taut band   a tight, rubber-band-like knot in the muscles.

T cell   a lymphocyte responsible for immunologic memory.

temporomandibular joint (TMJ) dysfunction syndrome   pain in the jaw joint associated with localized myofascial discomfort.

tender point   an area of tenderness in the muscles, tendons, bony prominences, or fat pads.

tendon   structure that attaches muscle to bone.

thalamus   an oval mass of gray matter in the brain that receives signals from nerve tracts in the spinal cord.

thyroid   a gland in the neck that makes a hormone that helps to regulate the body's metabolism.

Tietze's syndrome   another term for costochondritis (see above).

tinnitus   ringing in the ears.

titer   amount of a substance.

toxic oil syndrome   a form of eosinophilia myalgic syndrome (see above) caused by adulterated cooking oil.

tricyclic   a family of antidepressant drugs such as Elavil that relieve depression, promote restful sleep, relax muscles, and raise the pain threshold.

trigger point   an area of muscle that, when touched, triggers a reaction of discomfort.

tryptophan   an amino acid that can be broken down to serotonin.

urinalysis   analyzing a urine sample under the microscope.

vaginismus   tightness of the vaginal muscles, which prevents or limits penetration during sexual intercourse.

vasculitis   inflammation of the blood vessels.

vertigo   malfunction of the vestibular (balance center) of the ear, producing a sensation that everything around you is in motion.

visceral hyperalgesia   pain amplification mediated by the parasympathetic nervous system thought to cause irritable bowel and ulcer-like symptoms.

vocational rehabilitation   training someone for an occupation, which takes into account the person's educational background and physical skills, as well as his or her handicaps or impairments.

vulvodynia   pain in the female genital area when infection, cancer, stricture, or inflammation has been ruled out.

yeast   a type of fungus.

Appendix 3
Fibromyalgia: A Complementary Medicine Doctor's Perspective

By Soram Singh Khalsa, M.D.

Soram Singh Khalsa, M.D., is a board-certified internist and past chairman of the Executive Steering Committee of the Complementary Medicine Program at Cedars-Sinai Medical Center in Los Angeles. He currently is the medical director of the East West Medical Research Institute. Over the past two and a half decades, he has broadened his training both in the United States and abroad by staying on the leading edge of therapeutics using homeopathy, acupuncture, and phytotherapeutics, which he integrates into his traditional practice of internal medicine. A graduate of Yale University, Dr. Khalsa is a founding member of the American Holistic Medical Association, and the American Academy of Medical Acupuncture. Dr. Khalsa may be reached at his website www.khalsamedical.com.

I appreciate this opportunity to present the complementary medicine clinician's perspective on the treatment of fibromyalgia. Complementary medicine is being used by an increasing percentage of Americans. In an article published in the *New England Journal of Medicine* in 1993, Dr. David Eisenberg stated that approximately one in three people in America had obtained treatment using complementary medicine over the course of a single year. A subsequent study by Dr. Eisenberg published in 1998, indicated that over the preceding seven years there had been a 47 percent increase in total visits to alternative medicine practitioners. This study shows that more and more Americans are using the modalities of complementary medicine, and there is increased coverage of this form of medicine in magazines and newspapers throughout the country.

Complementary medicine includes many of the modalities mentioned in this book, including chiropractic, osteopathy, nutritional medicine, herbology and homeopathy, and many others. In my practice of medicine, I often use the term *functional medicine* to describe what I do. The Institute of Functional Medicine has created a formal definition: "Functional medicine is a field of healthcare focused on the assessment and early intervention into the improvement of physiological, cognitive/emotional, and physical functioning." The objective is to assess individual uniqueness and implement programs using diet, lifestyle practices, and activities tailored to the person's need to promote health, resilience, vitality, and performance. There is no illness more relevant to these goals than fibromyalgia.

The primary focus of complementary medicine is the concept of the spectrum of health (see Figure 17). At one end of the spectrum of health are diseases with pathology in which tissue change and/or organ damage are detectable with blood tests, X-rays, and pathology reports. At the opposite end of the spectrum is optimal well-being. Between these extremes is a transition zone. In the transition zone, organs show no signs of pathology, yet a patient can have many symptoms. In this zone, organs begin to lose their functional reserve and do not function ideally. The goal of functional medicine is to understand where patients fall on this spectrum. Almost always, unless fibromyalgia is a component of a pathologic disease such as lupus, patients with fibromyalgia fall in the central transition zone of this spectrum of health.

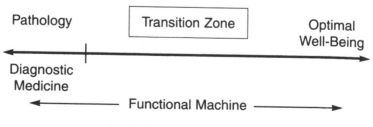

Fig. 17 *The spectrum of health*

Many medical problems in this central zone include an interaction of dysfunctions of the immune, endocrine, neurologic, hepatic, and gastrointestinal systems. As this book clearly points out, with its interaction between the endocrine, immune, and autonomic nervous system, fibromyalgia is one such illness.

A new diagnostic tool called Computerized Regulation Thermography, was approved in 1998 by the FDA for the evaluation of inflammatory conditions. This tool allows us to look indirectly at autonomic innervation of all the major organs in the body, and determine which organs are most dysregulated. With this modality we are now able to target our support for these underlying organs with greater accuracy.

In functional medicine, we use the concept put forth by Dr. Leo Galland that there are antecedents, including genetic susceptibility, aging, and nutritional insufficiency, combined with specific triggers in our environment that include not only a physical trauma but also food antigens and toxins, xenobiotics, endotoxins, and psychological or physiologic stress. This combination of antecedents and triggers leads to the mediators, discussed in this book, that produce the inflammatory response. These include the inflammatory cytokines, including cyclooxygenase and lipoxygenase, as well as the nitric acid cytokines. These inflammatory mediators directly affect the intermediate organs of the nervous, immune, gastrointestinal, and hepatic systems. They also produce oxidative stress, which further influences these systems. This creates dysfunction in these systems, which results in the symptoms that we see in the muscular, nervous, and endocrine systems in fibromyalgia.

Dr. Wallace is correct in saying that as yet there are no formal studies proving the relationship of dysfunctional gastrointestinal function and hepatic detoxification to fibromyalgia. We do know, however, that increased permeability of the lining of the gastrointestinal tract (sometimes called leaky gut) is a factor in some autoimmune illnesses, including ankylosing spondylitis and rheumatoid arthritis. Many factors, including abnormal intestinal flora, can contribute to this increased permeability. Every day in my practice and in those of hundreds of my colleagues who practice as I do, we find abnormalities in these functions in patients with fibromyalgia. By correcting them, we frequently achieve major improvements in the patient's symptoms. Formal studies to document and prove this are starting to be done. Indeed one recent study has shown a connection between small bowel bacterial over-growth and fibromyalgia.

Herbs, acupuncture, and homeopathy must be understood as agents used to reduce the dysfunction of the intermediate organs. Using them in combination can result in a potentiation of their effects, a result superior to that achieved by any one of the modalities alone. Although acupuncture is commonly thought of for its use in pain control, its major use is in supporting organ function. Vitamins and other nutritional cofactors including a variety of phytonutrients are used to help modify the inflammatory process, reduce intermediate inflammatory cytokines, and reduce the activity of the arachidonic acid cascade, thereby leading to reduced inflammation and the relief of pain. Specific nutritional cofactors, including the omega-3 family of fatty acids (as found in flaxseed oil and fish oil) need to be studied for their role in suppressing T helper-1 cell production, thereby ameliorating the cause of inflammation. One such clinical trial has been published, showing the use of eicosapentaenoic acid (EPA) and docosahexaenoic acid (DHA) in inflammatory disorders such as inflammatory bowel disease, rheumatoid arthritis, and psoriasis. More studies need to be done to see if these nutritional cofactors can be equally effective in modulating inflammation in fibromyalgia. In my clinical experience, they can indeed be useful.

Fortunately since the first edition of this book, controlled trials using complementary therapies are starting to be done for fibromyalgia. In one exciting pilot trial done at the Functional Medicine Research Center in Gig Harbor, Washington, a complex medical food designed for the clinical management of inflammatory conditions produced significant benefit for fibromyalgia patients, including improvement in mental functioning, a significant decrease in tender points, and a substantial improvement in grip strength and physical symptoms. This complex food contained vitamins, minerals, antioxidants, and other micronutrients as well as the phytonutrients curcumin, rosemary extract, rutin, ginger, and D-limonene. It was theorized by the authors of this article that these phytochemicals and nutrients probably worked by having a modulating effect on subclinical inflammatory processes, including effects on interleukin-1, tumor necrosis factor, and cyclooxygenase.

Another recent article from the complementary program at the University of Maryland School of Medicine, concluded that there is moderately strong evidence that acupuncture may be effective for treating fibromyalgia.

Other studies have shown that individual dietary supplements including melatonin, chlorella, malic acid, and SAMe can be helpful in some fibromyalgia patients.

In several other articles, a strict vegan diet had beneficial effects on fibromyalgia symptoms including decreased joint stiffness and pain as well as improvements in the patient's self-experienced health.

Because the basal autonomic state of patients with fibromyalgia is characterized by increased sympathetic and decreased parasympathetic tones, it is no surprise that some recent studies have proven that biofeedback can be effective in some fibromyalgia patients. Other treatments including spa treatments, massage, hypnotherapy, and meditation can be effective for similar reasons.

Additional areas of interest for research in complementary medicine include the role that female hormones and their changes during peri-menopause, as well as the role that heavy metals and environmental pollutants may have in contributing to fibromyalgia. The latter have been shown to have an almost certain link to autoimmune diseases including lupus.

In my practice with the very ill fibromyalgia patient, I endeavor to develop an overview of all the antecedents, triggers, and mediators involved, and to evaluate the functional integrity of the gastrointestinal, hepatic, and antioxidant systems of the body. By targeting therapy to the dysfunctional organs and modifying the specific triggers in the patient's environment, very gratifying clinical results are usually obtained.

By using this integrated approach to improving the functioning of the body's organ systems, there is one very interesting surprise. Most of us are familiar with the concept of psychosomatic influence, whereby the mind can produce effects in the body. In my many years of treating fibromyalgia, I have observed the somatopsychic effects of complementary medical treatment. Specifically in the case of fibromyalgia, I often find that by strengthening organ function through the modalities mentioned above, a patient's mental and emotional states can dramatically improve. Commonly in my practice, patients are able to reduce or sometimes eliminate their use of psychotropic medications as their physiology improves. This idea of somatopsychic effects needs to be studied much further. It has been observed frequently by many of my colleagues as well. Indeed in the above medical food study, mental functioning as assessed by the SF-36 questionnaire was significantly improved along with the other symptoms of fibromyalgia.

One of the problems in studying disorders in the transition zone of the spectrum of health is that there is no specific organ pathology. Rather, problems in this area are usually a complex of multiple organ system dysfunctions without disease. It is for this reason that the traditional medical study, which looks at only one variable and its effect on a target symptom, tends not to show the effectiveness of a single nutritional, herbal, or other complementary interaction. In the functional medicine approach to illness, several therapies are usually administered at once. For this reason, I believe that only outcome studies will be able to document the clinical effectiveness of most complementary forms of therapy. Medical outcome studies are more focused on function than on disease. This is very important in illnesses such as fibromyalgia. Specifically, medical outcome studies look at physical functioning, physical role, bodily pain, general health and vitality, and social functioning, as well as emotional role and mental health. These are the most important considerations in illnesses such as fibromyalgia, rather than simply looking at a result of one laboratory study, which the double blind, crossover, placebo-controlled model of most current medical studies facilitates. Most of the studies that I have cited above are indeed such medical outcome studies.

More and more we are seeing a new medical world where collaboration between traditional medical doctors and complementary medical doctors, as well as the variety of other complementary practitioners, including chiropractors, acupuncturists, herbologists, homeopaths, and osteopaths, will facilitate patient outcomes. In this way, we can continue to prove and document, in ways acceptable to all practitioners and patients, the effectiveness of these complementary modalities and the benefits of their integration with traditional medicine for the patient's health. After all, that is why all healthcare practitioners have embarked on their profession. This cooperation among practitioners and integration of care will lead to the improvement of patient outcomes and, in my opinion, will be especially effective in transitional zone illnesses, of which fibromyalgia is a most important example.

Index